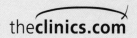

NEUROIMAGING CLINICS

OF NORTH AMERICA

Spinal Imaging: Overview and Update

Guest Editor

MAJDA M. THURNHER, MD

Consulting Editors

MAURICIO CASTILLO, MD, FACR
SURESH K. MUKHERJI, MD

February 2007 • Volume 17 • Number 1

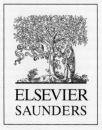

ELSEVIER
SAUNDERS

An imprint of Elsevier, Inc
PHILADELPHIA LONDON TORONTO MONTREAL SYDNEY TOKYO

W.B. SAUNDERS COMPANY

A Division of Elsevier Inc.

1600 John F. Kennedy Boulevard • Suite 1800 • Philadelphia, Pennsylvania 19103-2899

http://www.theclinics.com

NEUROIMAGING CLINICS Volume 17, Number 1
February 2007 ISSN 1052-5149, ISBN-13: 978-1-4160-4335-5, ISBN-10: 1-4160-4335-7

Editor: Lisa Richman

The ideas and opinions expressed in *Neuroimaging Clinics* do not necessarily reflect those of the Publisher. The Publisher does not assume any responsibility for any injury and/or damage to persons or property arising out of or related to any use of the material contained in this periodical. The reader is advised to check the appropriate medical literature and the product information currently provided by the manufacturer of each drug to be administered to verify the dosage, the method and duration of administration, or contraindications. It is the responsibility of the treating physician or other health care professional, relying on independent experience and knowledge of the patient, to determine drug dosages and the best treatment for the patient. Mention of any product in this issue should not be construed as endorsement by the contributors, editors, or the Publisher of the product or manufacturers' claims.

Neuroimaging Clinics (ISSN 1052-5149) is published quarterly by Elsevier Inc., 360 Park Avenue South, New York, NY 10010-1710. Months of issue are February, May, August, and November. Business and editorial offices: 1600 John F. Kennedy Blvd., Suite 1800, Philadelphia, PA 19103-2899. Business and editorial offices: 6277 Sea Harbor Drive, Orlando, FL 32887-4800. Periodicals postage paid at New York, NY, and additional mailing offices. Subscription prices are USD 218 per year for US individuals, USD 336 per year for US institutions, USD 112 per year for US students and residents, USD 252 per year for Canadian individuals, USD 413 per year for Canadian institutions, USD 302 per year for international individuals, USD 413 per year for international institutions and USD 151 per year for Canadian and foreign students and residents. To receive student/resident rate, orders must be accompanied by name of affiliated institution, date of term, and the *signature* of program/residency coordinator on institution letterhead. Orders will be billed at individual rate until proof of status is received. Foreign air speed delivery is included in all *Clinics* subscription prices. All prices are subject to change without notice. POSTMASTER: Send address changes to *Neuroimaging Clinics*, Elsevier Periodicals Customer Service, 6277 Sea Harbor Drive, Orlando, FL 32887-4800. **Customer Service: 1-800-654-2452 (US). From outside of the US, call (+1) 407-345-4000. E-mail: hhspcs@harcourt.com.**

Reprints. For copies of 100 or more, of articles in this publication, please contact the Commercial Reprints Department, Elsevier Inc., 360 Park Avenue South, New York, New York 10010-1710. Tel.: (+1) 212-633-3813; Fax: (+1) 212-462-1935; E-mail: reprints@elsevier.com.

Neuroimaging Clinics is covered by *Excerpta Medica/EMBASE*, the RSNA Index of Imaging Literature, Index Medicus, MEDLINE/MEDLARS, SciSearch, Research Alert, and Neuroscience Citation Index.

Printed in the United States of America.

GOAL STATEMENT

The goal of *Neuroimaging Clinics of North America* is to keep practicing radiologists and radiology residents up to date with current clinical practice in radiology by providing timely articles reviewing the state of the art in patient care.

ACCREDITATION

The *Neuroimaging Clinics of North America* is planned and implemented in accordance with the Essential Areas and Policies of the Accreditation Council for Continuing Medical Education (ACCME) through the joint sponsorship of the University of Virginia School of Medicine and Elsevier. The University of Virginia School of Medicine is accredited by the ACCME to provide continuing medical education for physicians.

The University of Virginia School of Medicine designates this educational activity for a maximum of 60 *AMA PRA Category 1 Credits*™. Physicians should only claim credit commensurate with the extent of their participation in the activity.

The American Medical Association has determined that physicians not licensed in the US who participate in this CME activity are eligible for *AMA PRA Category 1 Credits*™.

Credit can be earned by reading the text material, taking the CME examination online at http://www.theclinics.com/home/cme, and completing the evaluation. After taking the test, you will be required to review any and all incorrect answers. Following completion of the test and evaluation, your credit will be awarded and you may print your certificate.

FACULTY DISCLOSURE/CONFLICT OF INTEREST

The University of Virginia School of Medicine, as an ACCME accredited provider, endorses and strives to comply with the Accreditation Council for Continuing Medical Education (ACCME) Standards of Commercial Support, Commonwealth of Virginia statutes, University of Virginia policies and procedures, and associated federal and private regulations and guidelines on the need for disclosure and monitoring of proprietary and financial interests that may affect the scientific integrity and balance of content delivered in continuing medical education activities under our auspices.

The University of Virginia School of Medicine requires that all CME activities accredited through this institution be developed independently and be scientifically rigorous, balanced and objective in the presentation/discussion of its content, theories and practices.

All authors/editors participating in an accredited CME activity are expected to disclose to the readers relevant financial relationships with commercial entities occurring within the past 12 months (such as grants or research support, employee, consultant, stock holder, member of speakers bureau, etc.). The University of Virginia School of Medicine will employ appropriate mechanisms to resolve potential conflicts of interest to maintain the standards of fair and balanced education to the reader. Questions about specific strategies can be directed to the Office of Continuing Medical Education, University of Virginia School of Medicine, Charlottesville, Virginia.

The authors/editors listed below have identified no professional/financial affiliations for themselves or their spouse/partner:

Hortensia Alvarez, MD; Michael Augustin, MD; Walter H. Backes, PhD; Fabiola Cartes-Zumelzu, MD; Mauricio Castillo, MD (Consulting Editor); Denis Ducreux, MD, PhD; David Facon, MD; Pierre Fillard, PhD; Massimo Gallucci, MD; Carlo Gandolfo, MD; Joachim M. Gilsbach, MD, PhD; John D. Grimme, MD; Franz J. Hans, MD, PhD; Michael V. Krasnokutsky, MD; Timo Krings, MD, PhD; Pierre Lasjuanias, MD, PhD; Jean-François Lepeintre, MD; Nicola Limbucci, MD; Pavel V. Maly, MD, PhD; Luigi Manfre; Giovanni Morana, MD; Christina Mueller-Mang, MD; Michael Mull, MD; Robbert J. Nijenhuis, MD; Augustin Ozanne, MD; Amalia Paonessa, MD; Paul M. Parizel, MD, PhD; Marcel Philipp, MD; Marcus H. T. Reinges, MD; Jerome Renoux, MD; Lisa Richman (Acquisitions Editor); Georges Rodesch, MD, PhD; Andrea Rossi, MD; Alessandra Splendiani, MD; Pia C. Sundgren, MD, PhD; Marc Tadié, MD; Armin K. Thron, MD, PhD; Majda M. Thurnher, MD (Guest Editor); Paolo Tortori-Donati, MD; Anja Van Campenhout, MD; Luc Van Den Hauwe, MD; and, A. Talia Vertinsky, MD.

The authors listed below have identified the following professional/financial affiliations for themselves or their spouse/partner:

Roland Bammer, PhD serves as a consultant for Endius, Inc., and is a patent holder with GE Healthcare. **Johan Van Goethem, MD, PhD** is a consultant for Aimmer Spine.

Disclosure of Discussion of non-FDA approved uses for pharmaceutical products and/or medical devices.

The University of Virginia School of Medicine, as an ACCME provider, requires that all authors/editors identify and disclose any "off label" uses for pharmaceutical products and/or for medical devices. The University of Virginia School of Medicine recommends that each reader fully review all the available data on new products or procedures prior to instituting them with patients.

TO ENROLL

To enroll in the Neuroimaging Clinics of North America Continuing Medical Education program, call customer service at 1-800-654-2452 or sign up online at *http://www.theclinics.com/home/cme*. The CME program is available to subscribers for an additional annual fee of USD 175.

SPINAL IMAGING: OVERVIEW AND UPDATE

CONSULTING EDITORS

MAURICIO CASTILLO, MD, FACR
Professor and Chief, Section of Neuroradiology, Department of Radiology, University of North Carolina School of Medicine, Chapel Hill, North Carolina

SURESH K. MUKHERJI, MD
Professor and Chief, Neuroradiology and Head and Neck Radiology; Professor, Radiology and Otolaryngology Head and Neck Surgery; and Associate Fellowship Program Director, Department of Radiology, University of Michigan Health System, Ann Arbor, Michigan

GUEST EDITOR

MAJDA M. THURNHER, MD
Department of Radiology, Neuroradiology Section, Medical University of Vienna, A-1090 Vienna, Austria

CONTRIBUTORS

HORTENSIA ALVAREZ, MD
Service de Neuroradiologie Diagnostique et Thérapeutique, Hôspital de Bicetre, France

MICHAEL AUGUSTIN, MD
Department of Radiology, Medical University of Graz, Graz, Austria

WALTER H. BACKES, PhD
Department of Radiology, University Hospital Maastricht, Maastricht, The Netherlands

ROLAND BAMMER, PhD
Stanford University, Department of Radiology, Lucas Center, Stanford, California

FABIOLA CARTES-ZUMELZU, MD
Department of Radiology, Neuroradiology Section, Medical University of Vienna, Waehringer Guertel 18-20, A-1090 Vienna, Austria

MAURICIO CASTILLO, MD, FACR
Professor and Chief, Section of Neuroradiology, Department of Radiology, University of North Carolina School of Medicine, Chapel Hill, North Carolina

DENIS DUCREUX, MD, PhD
Department of Neuroradiology, CHU de Bicetre, Paris XI University; LIMEC, INSERM UMR 788, Le Kremlin Bicetre, France

DAVID FACON, MD
Department of Neuroradiology, CHU de Bicêtre, Paris XI University, Le Kremlin-Bicêtre, France

PIERRE FILLARD, PhD
Asclepios Research Project, Sophia Antipolis, France

MASSIMO GALLUCCI, MD
Professor, Department of Radiology, University of L'Aquila, S. Salvatore Hospital, L'Aquila, Italy

CARLO GANDOLFO, MD
Staff Neuroradiologist, Department of Pediatric Neuroradiology, G. Gaslini Children's Hospital, Genoa, Italy

JOACHIM M. GILSBACH, MD, PhD
Department of Neurosurgery, University Hospital Aachen, Aachen, Germany

JOHN D. GRIMME, MD
Fellow in Neuroradiology, Department of Radiology, University of North Carolina School of Medicine, Chapel Hill, North Carolina

FRANZ J. HANS, MD
Department of Neurosurgery, University Hospital
Aachen, Aachen, Germany

MICHAEL V. KRASNOKUTSKY, MD
Stanford University, Department of Radiology,
Lucas Center, Stanford, California

TIMO KRINGS, MD, PhD
Department of Neuroradiology, University
Hospital Aachen, Aachen, Germany; Service de
Neuroradiologie Diagnostique et Thérapeutique,
Hôspital de Bicetre, France; and Department of
Neurosurgery, University Hospital Aachen,
Aachen, Germany

PIERRE L. LASJAUNIAS, MD, PhD
Service de Neuroradiologie Diagnostique
et Thérapeutique, Hôspital de Bicetre, France

JEAN-FRANÇOIS LEPEINTRE, MD
Department of Neurosurgery,
CHU de Bicêtre, Paris XI University,
Le Kremlin-Bicêtre, France

NICOLA LIMBUCCI, MD
Department of Radiology, University of L'Aquila,
S. Salvatore Hospital, L'Aquila, Italy

PAVEL V. MALY, MD, PhD
Associate Professor, Department of Radiology,
University Hospital MAS, University of Lund,
Malmoe, Sweden

GIOVANNI MORANA, MD
Staff Neuroradiologist, Department of Pediatric
Neuroradiology, G. Gaslini Children's Hospital,
Genoa, Italy

CHRISTINA MUELLER-MANG, MD
Department of Radiology, Neuroradiology
Section, Medical University of Vienna, Waehringer
Guertel 18-20, A-1090 Vienna, Austria

MICHAEL MULL, MD
Department of Neuroradiology, University
Hospital Aachen, Aachen, Germany

ROBBERT J. NIJENHUIS, MD
Department of Radiology, University Hospital
Maastricht, Maastricht, The Netherlands

AUGUSTIN OZANNE, MD
Department of Neuroradiology, CHU de Bicêtre,
Paris XI University, Le Kremlin-Bicêtre,
France

AMALIA PAONESSA, MD
Department of Neuroradiology, Loreto Nuovo
Hospital, Naples, Italy

PAUL M. PARIZEL, MD, PhD
Department of Radiology, University of Antwerp,
Edegem (Antwerp), Belgium

MARCEL PHILIPP, MD
Department of Radiology, Medical University
Vienna, Vienna, Austria

MARCUS H.T. REINGES, MD
Department of Neurosurgery, University Hospital
Aachen, Aachen, Germany

JEROME RENOUX, MD
Department of Neuroradiology, CHU de Bicêtre,
Paris XI University, Le Kremlin-Bicêtre, France

GEORGES RODESCH, MD, PhD
Service de Neuroradiologie Diagnostique et
Thérapeutique, Hôpital de Bicetre, France

ANDREA ROSSI, MD
Acting Head, Department of Pediatric
Neuroradiology, G. Gaslini Children's Hospital,
Genoa, Italy

ALESSANDRA SPLENDIANI, MD
Department of Radiology, University of L'Aquila,
S. Salvatore Hospital, L'Aquila, Italy

PIA C. SUNDGREN, MD, PhD
Professor of Radiology, Department of Radiology,
University of Michigan Health Systems,
Ann Arbor, Michigan

MARC TADIÉ, MD
Department of Neurosurgery, CHU de Bicêtre,
Paris XI University, Le Kremlin-Bicêtre,
France

ARMIN K. THRON, MD, PhD
Department of Neuroradiology, University
Hospital Aachen, Aachen, Germany

MAJDA M. THURNHER, MD
Department of Radiology, Neuroradiology
Section, Medical University of Vienna,
A-1090 Vienna, Austria

PAOLO TORTORI-DONATI, MD
Former Head (now retired), Department of
Pediatric Neuroradiology, G. Gaslini Children's
Hospital, Genoa, Italy

A. VAN CAMPENHOUT, MD
Department of Orthopaedics,
University Hospitals Leuven,
Pellenberg, Belgium

LUC VAN DEN HAUWE, MD
Department of Radiology, University of Antwerp,
Edegem (Antwerp), Belgium

JOHAN VAN GOETHEM, MD, PhD
Department of Radiology, University of Antwerp,
Edegem (Antwerp), Belgium; Department of
Radiology, AZ Nikolaas, Sint-Niklaas, Belgium

A. TALIA VERTINSKY, MD
Stanford University, Department of Radiology,
Lucas Center, Stanford, California

SPINAL IMAGING: OVERVIEW AND UPDATE

Volume 17 · Number 1 · February 2007

Contents

The complexity of the congenital anomalies of the spine can make the neuroradiologic diagnosis challenging. Knowledge of spinal embryology greatly helps in the understanding and classification of these anomalies. We use the classification devised by Tortori-Donati and Rossi and find it helpful from clinical and imaging standpoints. We believe that most patients who have known or suspected congenital spinal anomalies benefit from MR imaging.

In children, tumors of the spine are much rarer than intracranial tumors. They are classified into intramedullary, intradural-extramedullary, and extradural tumors. Magnetic resonance imaging provides crucial information regarding the extent, location, and internal structure of the mass, thus critically narrowing the differential diagnosis and guiding surgery.

Spinal cord diseases generally have distinctive clinical findings that reflect dysfunction of particular sensory or motor tracts. The abnormalities on MR images reflect the pathologic changes that occur in the affected pathways. The complexity and the wide spectrum of diseases affecting the spinal cord require a profound knowledge of neuropathology and exactly tuned imaging strategies. This article describes and illustrates the clinical and imaging characteristics in various demyelinating and infectious conditions of the spinal cord.

Spinal vascular diseases are rare and constitute only 1% to 2% of all vascular neurologic pathologies. In this article, the following vascular pathologies of the spine are described: spinal arterial infarcts, spinal cavernomas, and arteriovenous malformations (including perimedullary fistulae and glomerular arteriovenous malformations), and spinal dural arteriovenous fistulae. This article gives an overview about their imaging features on MRI, MR angiography, and digital subtraction angiography. Clinical differential diagnoses, the neurologic symptomatology, and the potential therapeutic approaches of these diseases, which might vary depending on the underlying pathologic condition, are given.

Approximately 30,000 spinal injuries occur in the United States every year. Injuries to the spine and its contents affect predominately young, healthy individuals and are a major cause of disability, with significant socioeconomic consequences. The main cause for spinal injuries is blunt trauma, most commonly caused by motor vehicle accidents, followed by falls and sport injuries. Already, in the initial evaluation of patients who have blunt trauma, multislice CT with two-dimensional (and threedimensional) reformatting is the method of choice. The liberal use of MR imaging is recommended to assess for injuries to soft tissue, the spine and its contents, intervertebral discs, and ligaments.

Degenerative disease of the spine is a definition that includes a wide spectrum of degenerative abnormalities. Degeneration involves bony structures and the intervertebral disk, although many aspects of spine degeneration are strictly linked because the main common pathogenic factor is identified in chronic overload. During life the spine undergoes continuous changes as a response to physiologic axial load. These age-related changes are similar to pathologic degenerative changes and are a common asymptomatic finding in adults and elderly persons. A mild degree of degenerative changes is paraphysiologic and should be considered pathologic only if abnormalities determine symptoms. Imaging allows complete evaluation of static and dynamic factors related to degenerative disease of the spine and is useful in diagnosing the different aspects of spine degeneration.

Scoliosis is a structural lateral curvature of the spine with a rotatory component. Imaging in scoliosis is important. Most cases of scoliosis are idiopathic, and imaging is used routinely in monitoring the changes of the deformity that take place during growth. Imaging is also crucial in determining the underlying etiology in non-idiopathic cases of scoliosis and is used in pre- and postoperative monitoring.

Damage to the spinal cord may be caused by a wide range of pathologies and generally results in profound functional disability. A reliable diagnostic workup of the spine is very important because even relatively small lesions in this part of the central nervous system can have a profound clinical impact. MR imaging has become the method of choice for the detection and diagnosis of many spine disorders. Various innovative MR imaging methods have been developed to improve neuroimaging, including better pulse sequences and new MR contrast parameters. These new "cutting-edge" technologies have the potential to impact profoundly the ease and confidence of spinal disease interpretation and offer a more efficient diagnostic workup of patients suffering from spinal disease.

Diffusion-weighted imaging and fractional anisotropy may be more sensitive than other conventional magnetic resonance imaging techniques to detect, characterize, and map the extent of spinal cord lesions. Fiber tracking offers the possibility of visualizing the integrity of white matter tracts surrounding some lesions, and this information may help in formulating a differential diagnosis and in planning biopsies or resection. Fractional anisotropy measurements may also play a role in predicting the outcome of patients who have spinal cord lesions. In this article, we address several conditions in which diffusion-weighted imaging and fiber tracking is known to be useful and speculate on others in which we believe these techniques will be useful in the near future.

ELSEVIER
SAUNDERS

NEUROIMAGING
CLINICS
OF NORTH AMERICA

Neuroimag Clin N Am 17 (2007) xiii

Foreword

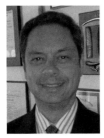
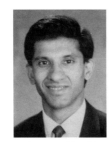

Mauricio Castillo,
MD, FACR

Suresh K. Mukherji, MD

Consulting Editors

Mauricio Castillo, MD, FACR
Division of Neuroradiology
Department of Radiology
University of North Carolina School of Medicine
Campus Box 7510
Chapel Hill, NC 27599-7510, USA

E-mail address:
castillo@med.unc.edu

Suresh K. Mukherji, MD
Department of Radiology, B2 A209-0030
University of Michigan Health System
1500 East Medical Center Drive
Ann Arbor, MI 48109-0030, USA

The readership of the *Neuroimaging Clinics* varies. Some readers like state-of-the-art and advanced articles, whereas others prefer reviews of more basic topics, and it is difficult as editors to satisfy both groups. For this issue of the Clinics, we have chosen a topic that, at first glance, appears to be geared toward the latter group of readers. Advances in spinal imaging have not been as drastic as those in brain imaging due to inherent difficulties encountered in this area, such as its relatively small size, motion, and its close bony surroundings. These factors have led to the relative lack of applications of diffusion, perfusion, spectroscopy, and functional imaging in the spine. As will be evident to readers after perusing this issue of the Clinics, some of these technical barriers are starting to be lifted while others have mostly disappeared. After reading the reviews by Drs. Ducreux and Bammer, it should be obvious to the readership that advances in spinal imaging are occurring, particularly in diffusion imaging and its applications. The remainder of this issue follows a more traditional division addressing what one may call "classic" topics in spinal imaging. These topics

include spinal dysraphisms, infections and demyelination, degenerative disease, and trauma. We consider these themes to be of great importance because they represent the majority of disorders that are seen in routine and daily clinical practice. Other less traditional reviews deal with tumors of the spine in children (which are of interest to pediatric neuroradiologists, pediatric radiologists, and others) and spinal instability. Imaging in spinal scoliosis is addressed by itself because it is a topic of daily importance that is rarely addressed in the neuroradiologic literature. Finally, we will be able to tell our residents and fellows where to find excellent information on this topic. Lastly, Dr. Krings has contributed with an article on imaging of spinal vascular diseases. This topic is also of great importance due to the advances in interventional neuroradiology as well as those in noninvasive vascular spinal imaging. Obviously, this issue is not all inclusive, and many topics are not found here as the format of the Clinics does not allow it. Nevertheless, we have no doubt that readers will find the articles published herein to be interesting and informative.

doi:10.1016/j.nic.2007.01.004

NEUROIMAGING CLINICS OF NORTH AMERICA

Neuroimag Clin N Am 17 (2007) xv–xvi

Preface

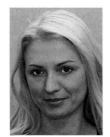

Majda M. Thurnher, MD
Guest Editor

Majda M. Thurnher, MD
Associate Professor of Radiology
Medical University of Vienna
Department of Radiology
Neuroradiology Section
Waehringer Guertel 18-20
A-1090 Vienna, Austria

E-mail address:
majda.thurnher@meduniwien.ac.at

Spinal cord research is based on studies of descriptive neuropathology, performed during the early nineteenth and twentieth centuries, with definitions of the basic nature of spinal cord diseases. Our understanding of the classification, diagnosis, pathogenesis, and treatment of spine and spinal cord diseases has recently begun to expand dramatically. The complexity of the different spinal compartments and the wide spectrum of diseases that affect the spine and spinal cord require precisely tuned imaging strategies.

MR imaging offers the advantages of multiplanar capabilities, physiologic and anatomic imaging, and some tissue specificity and has replaced other imaging modalities as the first choice in the evaluation of the spine. MR imaging has also become an integral part in the staging of primary and secondary tumors of the spine, as well as in guiding therapy, and is an excellent modality for follow-up.

A large gap between the promises of high-field MR imaging in evaluating spine disorders and the clinical reality characterizes the current literature. There are many advantages and challenges associated with clinical 3 T imaging of the spine. Despite the general lack of optimism about the usefulness of 3 T magnetic resonance in spinal cord imaging, the potential to obtain high-resolution images of the spinal cord in short scan times renders high-field imaging a powerful diagnostic tool for the future.

With this issue of *Neuroimaging Clinics of North America*, we aim to (1) illustrate the imaging characteristics in different pathologic conditions of the spinal column and spinal cord and (2) update the reader about current imaging techniques in the evaluation of the spinal column and spinal cord. In addition, articles in this issue propose simple algorithms to aid in deciding which patients would be ideally treated medically and which patients would benefit from spine surgery.

The only approach to improvement of spinal imaging is the concept of a "big vision, small steps." For many years, the big vision of neuroradiologists

doi:10.1016/j.nic.2007.01.005

has been to raise the quality and diagnostic significance of spinal imaging to the level of brain imaging. New technical steps and the recent results of published studies have increased our confidence that significant improvements will materialize in the clinical routine.

I would like to express my deep gratitude to all of the authors and my colleagues and friends in Europe and the United States for their effort and expertise in preparing this issue and their consistent dedication to the effort to improve spinal cord imaging.

NEUROIMAGING
CLINICS
OF NORTH AMERICA

Neuroimag Clin N Am 17 (2007) xvii

Dedication

To my son Alexander.

doi:10.1016/j.nic.2007.03.007

NEUROIMAGING
CLINICS
OF NORTH AMERICA

Neuroimag Clin N Am 17 (2007) 1–16

ELSEVIER
SAUNDERS

Congenital Anomalies of the Spine

John D. Grimme, MD, Mauricio Castillo, MD, FACR*

- Embryology
- Pathology
  Open dysraphisms
  Closed dysraphisms with associated mass

Closed dysraphisms without associated mass
- Summary
- References

The spine is a complex anatomic structure that is formed by elaborate mechanisms. Congenital spinal anomalies tend to be complex, and their names and classification are often confusing. Although most congenital spinal anomalies present in the newborn period, some of them (particularly the so-called "occult" or "closed" ones) may not be found until adulthood. Severe or "open" dysraphisms and those also affecting the development of the distal gastrointestinal and genitourinary tracts and of the lower extremities are generally rapidly diagnosed and may require immediate treatment to avoid complications. At least a basic understanding of the development of the spine is needed before attempting to interpret imaging studies of congenital spinal anomalies. We begin this article with a brief overview of spine development because discreet anomalies can generally be traced back to failure of specific embryologic mechanisms. We attempt to follow the classifications of these anomalies proposed by Tortori-Donati and Rossi [1,2] but have taken the liberty to insert our own points of view. Regardless of our opinion, the classification developed by Tortori-Donati and Rossi is a valid and valuable one. We believe that most congenital spinal anomalies are better portrayed with MR imaging than with any other imaging technique; therefore, the use of MR imaging is emphasized throughout this article. We address the more commonly encountered congenital anomalies involving the spine, with emphasis on dysraphisms and masses.

Embryology

During the first stage of embryologic development (called the "pre-neurulation" stage), the primitive streak forms on approximately day 17 and consists of a longitudinal primitive groove and a primitive node (Hensen's node) with a central pit at the presumptive cranial end (Fig. 1). These structures are located on the dorsal (chorionic) surface of the bilaminar embryonic disc. At this time, there is an invagination of cells near the primitive streak between the epiblast (future ectoderm) and the endoderm, forming the mesoderm. This process is called gastrulation. The mesoderm cells that travel through the primitive pit and migrate cranially form the notochordal process (the notochord process initially is a hollow tube called the "notochordal canal"), which parallels the streak. The ventral aspect of the notochordal process fuses to the subjacent endoderm and opens ventrally from the region of the primitive pit, effectively unzipping itself and allowing for a transient communication between the yolk sac and amniotic (ventral surface) cavities. Anomalies at this stage include the so-called "split notochord" anomalies, of which the most common is diastematomyelia. The least common anomalies are intraspinal enteric cysts and fistulas. The open

Department of Radiology, 3324 Old Infirmary, CB # 7510, University of North Carolina School of Medicine, Chapel Hill, NC 27599-7510, USA
* Corresponding author.
E-mail address: castillo@med.unc.edu (M. Castillo).

1052-5149/07/$ – see front matter. Published by Elsevier Inc.   doi:10.1016/j.nic.2006.11.002
neuroimaging.theclinics.com

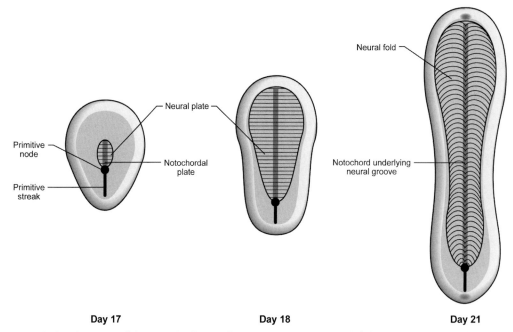

Day 17	Day 18	Day 21

Fig. 1. Early development of the neural tube. At day 17, the primitive streak forms distal to the node. Cephalad to these structures is the neural plate; ventral to them the notochordal plate. At day 18 the plates enlarge, and by day 21 they extend from one fetal pole to the other. At this time the neural plate begins to curve dorsally and form the neural folds.

neural tube then flattens and is contiguous with the embryonic endoderm as the notochordal plate. At approximately day 23, the notochordal plate detaches from the neural tube (embryonic ectoderm) and is converted in the process to the definitive solid structure known as the notochord (by obliteration of the notochordal cavity) (Fig. 2).

The notochord does not form elements of the spinal column; however, it plays an important role in the induction of the vertebral bodies (via the para-axial mesoderm) and of the neural tube. Likely in response to induction from the underlying notochordal plate and prechordal plate, a focal area of thickening appears in the surface of the epiblast, called the neural plate. While the cranial portion of the neural plate forms the brain, the caudal portion, overlying the notochord, becomes the spinal cord.

The second stage of development is called "primary neurulation" (from day 17 to about day 28 of life) and is responsible for the formation of nearly 90% of the spinal cord. The caudal portion of the neural plate elongates rapidly from days 22 to 26, and there is a respective elongation of the underlying notochord. During this period, a groove forms along the central portion of the neural plate, and its lateral margins become thickened and raised. These thickened lateral margins are called the "neural crests." At these levels, a group of specialized cells (the neural crest cells) originate and later migrate ventrally to establish peripheral nerves and various mesodermal and vascular structures. The neural crests continue to fold in a concave fashion to meet in the midline and eventually close to form a tube-like structure (the "neural tube"). An increased gradient of bone morphogenic protein establishes the dorsal surface of the neural tube, while an increased gradient of sonic hedgehog gene locates the ventral aspect of the neural tube (therefore establishing the posterior and anterior surfaces of the spinal cord). The spine is established by the presence of repetitive segments called rhombomeres. The organization of these rhombomeres is highly preserved from lesser animals to human beings. These rhombomeres express a variety of genes whose presence aids in the organized development of the spine. Traditionally, the neural tube has been assumed to first fuse in its center and then to extend this closure cephalad and caudally in a zipper-like fashion. This mechanism fails to explain the presence of open spinal dysraphisms in sites other then the extremes of the neural tube. Thus, it is likely that neural tube closure occurs simultaneously at several sites also in a zipper-like manner. From this explanation, it is obvious that failure of primary neurulation results in "open" dysraphisms, which are a group of disorders in which a portion

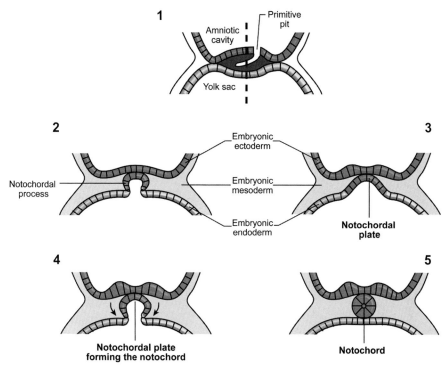

Fig. 2. Diagram illustrating notochordal development. (*Top*) (*1*): sagittal view through the embryonic disc shows the dorsal (amniotic) and ventral (yolk sac) surfaces of the disc. Note primitive pit and its extension ventrally. (*Bottom*) Four images are transverse sections at the level of the *dashed line* in top drawing. (*2*) The ventral aspect invaginates into the disc to form the notochordal process. (*3*) The notochordal process forms the plate. (*4*) The edges of plate approximate each other to fuse in the midline. (*5*) When the edges fuse completely, a round tube (notochord) is formed and is located between the amniotic and chorionic surfaces of the embryo.

of the neural tube remains exposed and visible (the most common of these disorders is the myelomeningocele).

Once closure of the neural tube commences, it detaches itself from the overlying ectoderm in a process called "disjunction." Disjunction may occur before its appropriate time (so-called "premature disjunction") or late (so-called "incomplete disjunction"). A variety of disorders may arise from either of these two abnormal mechanisms.

The third and last stage in the development of the spine is called "secondary neurulation" and involves the formation of about 10% of the spine, all of it in the caudal-most region. In this process, the most important mechanism is that of "canalization and retrogressive differentiation." The distal-most notochord and neural tube merge inferiorly at the caudal cell mass. The undifferentiated cells in this mass give rise to the bones of the sacrum, coccyx, and probably the fifth lumbar vertebra. They induce cavitation of the distal neural tube until it contains only one central canal (canalization) (Fig. 3). This canalized tube regresses in a cephalad manner (ie, retrogressive differentiation), establishing the nerve roots and the conus medullaris.

Complete regression of its cells leaves behind a strand that is made off only pia and ependyma (the filum terminale). Incomplete closure of the central canal in the conus medullaris results in the presence of a terminal ventricle. Exaggerated retrogressive differentiation may be one cause responsible for the caudal regression (or agenesis) syndrome. Maldifferentiation of the caudal cell mass may also contribute to the development of sacro-coccygeal teratomas.

Pathology

Developmental errors can occur at any stage of embryogenesis, alone or in tandem. This can create confusion when making a neuroradiologic diagnosis. Rossi and Tortori-Donati and colleagues have written extensively on the classification of spinal dysraphisms, attempting to simplify this task and remove ambiguity [1,2]. They suggest that the initial classification should be made clinically by determining whether there is an open or closed spinal dysraphism (ie, whether the defect is open to the air, thus leaving the neural elements exposed and visible) or is covered by a layer of skin, which

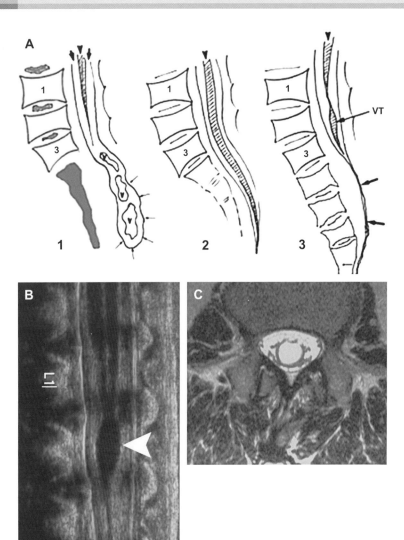

Fig. 3. Secondary neurulation and persistent ventriculus terminus. (*A*) (*1*) The primitive cell mass (*tiny arrows*) begins to be vacuolated (V) and joins the spina cord (*small arrows*) superiorly but is separated from the cord's central canal (*arrowhead*). (*2*) The canalized caudal cell mass joins the central canal (*arrowhead*) and assumes a more tubular shape. (*3*) The caudal cell mass undergoes retrogressive differentiation and leaves behind the filum terminal (*lower arrowhead*). The central canal (*superior arrowhead*) is contiguous inferiorly with the terminal ventricle (*long arrow*). (*B*) Sagittal sonogram shows a prominent terminal ventricle (*arrowhead*). (*C*) An axial T2-weighted image (different patient) shows an incidentally found large terminal ventricle.

would prevent the visualization of the neural elements [1,2]. If closed, the lesion can be further characterized by whether or not there is an associated mass. Clues as to the presence of an underlying closed dysraphisms may be found during the physical examination and include a midline dimple, dermal sinus, port wine stain, focal hirsutism, lower extremity deformities, and anal and genitourinary anomalies [3,4]. Spinal dysraphisms are often diagnosed prenatally by the presence of elevated maternal alpha fetoprotein in cases of open neural tube defects and by prenatal sonography and MR imaging [5–7]. In some cases, in utero surgical repair of the defect may be performed [8].

Open dysraphisms

Open spinal dysraphisms include myelomeningoceles, myeloceles, hemimyelomeningoceles, and hemimyeloceles, all of which have associated Chiari II malformations of varying degrees of severity. Myelomeningoceles account for nearly 99% of open spinal dysraphisms. In developing countries, the overall incidence of myelomeningocele is about 2 out of 1000 live births, whereas in industrialized nations and with the administration of preconception and prenatal maternal folates, their incidence has dropped to about 2 out of 10,000 live births. MR imaging and sonography permit for in utero diagnosis of myelomeningoceles (Fig. 4). Myelomeningoceles are usually easily diagnosed clinically by the presence of a large protruding mass containing the nonneurulated neural tissue called a "placode." In these patients, a prominent ventral subarachnoid cerebral spinal fluid–filled space pushes the placode away from the surface of the skin (Fig. 5). Myeloceles also have an exposed

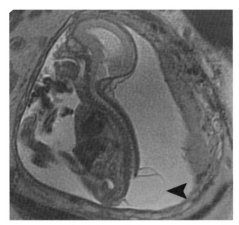

Fig. 4. In utero T2-weighted MR HASTE image shows a large lumbo-sacral myelomeningocele (*arrowhead*) and hydrocephalus.

placode; however, there is no associated expansion of the subarachnoid space and the placode remains flush with the cutaneous surface. Both defects are usually found at the lumbosacral level but may occur elsewhere in the spine. Accompanying all open defects is an incomplete migration of the para-axial mesenchyme, resulting in a bony spinal defect (spina bifida) and significant muscle atrophy, both of which contribute to the development of scoliosis. This is the origin of the term "spinal bifida aperta," which is no longer used. In the rare case of tandem errors in gastrulation and neurulation, there is a diastematomyelia, and one of the hemicords is contained in a myelomeningocele or a myelocele resulting in a hemimyelomeningocele or hemimyelocele (both rare anomalies). MR imaging is the modality of choice to preoperatively assess the

components of these malformations, to define the anatomic relationship of the placode with the underlying nerve roots, and to search for associated abnormalities. Many surgeons repair the dysraphisms without obtaining an imaging study of the spine. Some type of imaging study of the brain is needed to exclude the presence of hydrocephalus (found in 75% of patients with open dysraphisms), which may be shunted at the time of the spinal repair.

In open dysraphisms, typically there is a low-lying dysplastic spinal cord, and the placode forms the posterior wall of the defect. In the case of the myelomeningocele, ventral to the placode there is a dilated subarachnoid space, through which the nerve roots traverse. The nerve roots arise from the ventral placode, which is the nontubulated outer surface of the cord. The conus medullaris is not normally formed, and imaging of the entire spine is needed to exclude the presence of a cord cavity (syringohydromyelia) or other defects, such as diastematomyelia.

Although one of the surgical goals is to untether the placode, reform it, and replace it in the native spinal canal, most placodes remain tethered to the site of repair. Therefore, postoperative imaging is performed to search not only for the status of the placode but also for other complications, such as developing hydromyelia, constriction dural rings at the site of grafting and repair, epidermoids and dermoids, ischemia of the cord, and diastematomyelia [1,2,9,10].

Closed dysraphisms with associated mass

We begin this discussion by addressing closed dysraphic states that have associated back masses. These

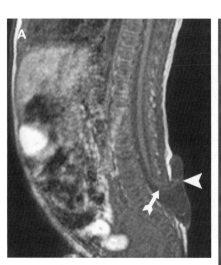

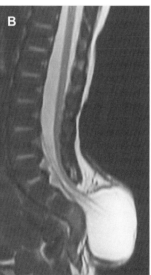

Fig. 5. (*A*) Sagittal T1-weighted MR image shows lumbosacral myelomeningocele. The cord (*arrow*) extends into the fluid-filled cyst and terminates in a placode (*arrowhead*). (*B*) In a different patient, a sagittal T2-weighted image shows the CSF-filled sac containing a dysplastic cord. (*Courtesy of A. Rossi, MD, Genoa, Italy.*)

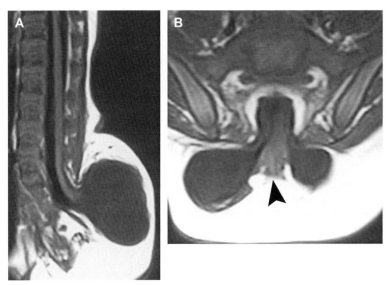

Fig. 6. (A) Sagittal T1-weighted MR image shows a CSF-filled sac containing neural elements. The sac protrudes posteriorly and is covered by fat and skin in this lipomyelomeningocele. (B) Axial T1-weighted image in a different patient showing the placode (*arrowhead*) lying outside of the location of the native spinal canal and contiguous with a lipoma. There are CSF-filled sacs herniating on both sides of the placode. (*Courtesy of* A. Rossi, Genoa, MD, Italy.)

include lipomyeloceles, lipomyelomeningoceles, meningoceles, and myelocystoceles. Lipomyeloceles and lipomyelomeningoceles also occur secondary to abnormal neurulation, where dysjunction occurs prematurely and allows primitive mesenchymal cells to migrate into the neural tube. When these cells reach the placode, they are induced to form adipose tissues. The result is the formation of a lipoma that traverses the bifid bony posterior elements and is contiguous with the epidural and subcutaneous fat. If the placode–lipoma complex remains within the spinal canal, the abnormality is called a lipomeningocele (analogous to the meningocele); if it lies outside of the confines of the spinal canal because the ventral subarachnoid space is expanded, it is called a lipomyelomeningocele (analogous to the myelomeningocele) (Figs. 6 and 7) [1,2,9].

A meningocele is a rare anomaly that manifests as a herniation of meninges through a neural foramen laterally or through a vertebral or sacral defect anteriorly or posteriorly [1,11,12]. The herniated sac consists of an outer layer of dura and an inner arachnoid membrane and usually contains only CSF, although occasionally it may contain nerve roots, dysplastic tissues, or tumor [12]. Often, meningoceles are associated with systemic mesenchymal disorders, such as neurofibromatosis type 1 or Marfan syndrome, but can be seen in isolated forms (Fig. 8) [11]. Over 80% of meningoceles are posterior and in the lumbosacral spine, but they are occasionally found in the thoracic spine and

sacrum and may become large enough to cause symptoms from mass effect (Fig. 9) [11,12]. Spinal meningoceles are thought to be caused by failed closure of the neural tube in the neurulation stage of development and then gradually increase in

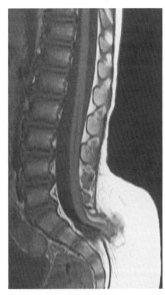

Fig. 7. Sagittal T1-weighted MR image shows a bone defect at the posterior sacral region into which the dysplastic cord extends. There is no CSF-filled sac, and the defect is covered by fat and skin in this lipomyelocele. (*Courtesy of* A. Rossi, MD, Genoa, Italy.)

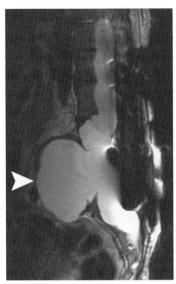

Fig. 8. Sagittal T2-weighted MR image in a patient who has neurofibromatosis type 1 shows a large pre-sacral meningocele (*arrowhead*).

size secondary to continual CSF pulsations [1,12]. Traditionally, these lesions were evaluated with plain radiographs, CT, and myelography, but MR imaging is now used most frequently because it allows for better characterization regarding its anatomic relationships and contents and may reveal other associated congenital lesions, such as genitourinary anomalies or spinal anomalies [12]. Eroded vertebral bodies, thinned vertebral arches, and expanded foramina are associated findings [11,13].

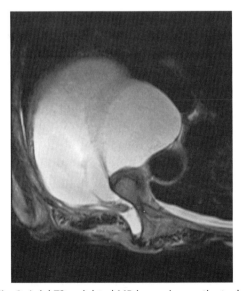

Fig. 9. Axial T2-weighted MR image in a patient who has neurofibromatosis type 1 shows a large lateral thoracic meningocele.

Spinal sonography in the newborn may show a cystic mass in an expanded spinal canal, with displacement of the spinal cord by the meningocele [13].

A myelocystocele is a large posterior meningocele that lies dorsal to a bony spina bifida and houses a large terminal syrinx (syringocele). The meningocele component is continuous with the subarachnoid space, and the syringocele is continuous with the ependymal canal. There is no communication between the two spaces [1,2]. This anomaly is rare.

Closed dysraphisms without associated mass

Closed dysraphisms without an associated mass include intradural, intramedullary, or filar lipomas and the tight filum terminale syndrome. Intradural and intramedullary lipomas lie within the dural sac, most commonly in the lumbosacral region, although they may be found at any level (Fig. 10A). At the level where they are contiguous with spinal cord, there is a placode, which often displaces the spinal cord away from the midline (Figs. 10B and 11). On MR imaging, lipomas should follow the signal intensity of subcutaneous fat in all sequences. Hyperintense T1 signal in a thickened filum terminale indicates a filar lipoma, which may be considered incidental if the patient does not have clinical signs of tethered cord syndrome and if the conus medullaris terminates at a normal level (never below the L2-L3 disc space) (Fig. 12). Filar lipomas are probably due to an anomaly of secondary neurulation (although some authors think that they are due to anomalies of retrogressive differentiation). The tight filum terminale syndrome develops due to abnormal differentiation of the secondary neural tube, causing the filum to be shortened and hindering the apparent ascent of the conus medullaris [1,2]. The filum can be considered to be thick when it measures more than 2 mm in diameter or is significantly thicker than the adjacent nerve roots. Symptomatic patients who have a thick filum and an abnormally low conus medullaris benefit from surgery.

Around the third week of gestation, when the cells from Hensen's node are proliferating and migrating, there may be a focal splitting of the notochord secondary to a persistent connection (canals of Kovalesky) between the endoderm and ectoderm [14–16]. Although there is debate over the exact mechanism, failure of midline integration of the notochord anlagen may result in a spectrum of rare anomalies with variable complexity. A dorsal enteric fistula is considered to be the most severe form, resulting in a persistent connection between the bowel and the posterior cutaneous surface, crossing between a duplicated spine [1,16]. Displaced endodermal tissue may be located anywhere along the path of the abnormal connection,

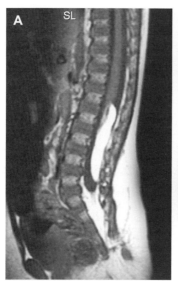
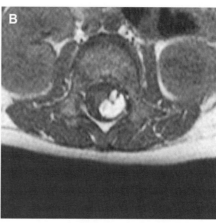

Fig. 10. (*A*) Sagittal T1-weighted MR image shows a lumbar intraspinal lipoma contiguous with the cord, which is slightly low in position. (*B*) Axial T1-weighted image shows that the lipoma is completely intradural. Note that the cord is flat (due to incomplete closure) at the level where the lipoma abuts it.

resulting in a neurenteric cyst, which may occur at any level of the spine but most commonly occurs in the lower cervical and upper thoracic regions. Neurenteric cysts may be intraspinal, intramedullary, or postvertebral but are often are prevertebral, located in the posterior mediastinum [15–18]. These cysts are lined by alimentary or respiratory epithelium and may produce mucus. Patients may present with signs of spinal cord compression from mass effect of the cyst or with meningitis in cases when the cyst ruptures into the subarachnoid space [17]. Multiple associated abnormalities have been described, including vertebral/spinal and cardiac anomalies, renal and limb dysgenesis, and various anomalies of the alimentary tract, such as partial duplications and fistulas [17,18]. "Split notochord syndrome" refers to associated vertebral anomalies, central nervous system abnormalities, and intestinal anomalies [14]. The imaging appearance is variable, depending on the location and severity of the abnormality. Depending on the protein content of the cystic material, the fluid may be

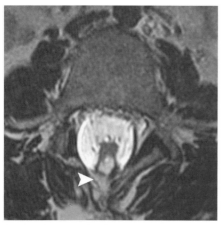

Fig. 11. Axial T2-weighted image shows continuation of subcutaneous lipoma (*arrowhead*) into the dorsal spinal canal. The lipoma insinuates itself into the cord, which did not close normally.

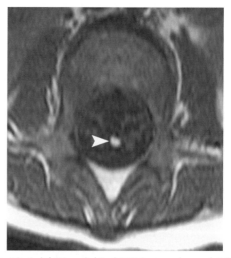

Fig. 12. Axial T1-weighted MR image shows fat (*arrowhead*) in the filum terminale, which is minimally thickened. In this patient, the conus medullaris terminated at a normal level, and the lipoma was considered to be incidental and not clinically significant.

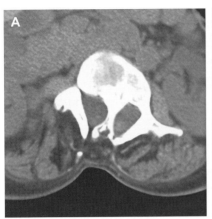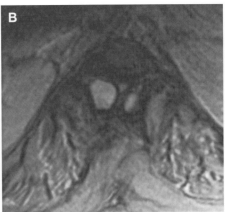

Fig. 13. (A) Axial CT shows a thick bone bar dividing the spinal canal (type 1 diastematomyelia). (B) Axial T2-weighted image in a similar case shows two distinct spinal canals separated by a low-intensity bar.

iso- to hyperintense on T1- and T2-weighted images [1]. These lesions generally do not enhance [1,18]. The sine qua non for a neurenteric cyst is a wide anterior spina bifida through which there is a direct communication between a cystic posterior mediastinal mass and the subarachnoid space [15].

If the notochord fails to fuse in the midline because of a persistent connection between the yolk sac and amniotic cavities and if there are cells from the primitive streak between the anlagen, two separate hemicords are formed. This is referred to as "diastematomyelia." The final outcome is dependent on progression or regression of the cells from the primitive streak. With progression, two separate neural plates are formed, and the hemicords eventually lie within two separate dural tubes, divided by a thick osteocartilaginous septum. This is called a "type I diastematomyelia" and is symptomatic due to tethering of the cord by the spur and often the presence of syringomyelia (Fig. 13). "Type II diastematomyelia" occurs when the cells of the primitive streak regress, with the end outcome being a single dural tube housing both hemicords, which may or may not be separated by a thin, nonrigid fibrous septum [1,2,19]. In the absence of a septum, these anomalies are nearly always asymptomatic but may come to clinical attention if a syrinx develops (Fig. 14).

Thought to be a result of focal areas of incomplete disjunction, dermal sinuses are tracts lined by squamous epithelium that connect the skin to deeper tissue layers and may extend to the intramedullary spinal cord space [20,21]. They occur in the dorsal midline at any level of the spine but are most commonly are found in the lumbosacral region [20–22]. The tracts may contain dermal and/or neuroglial elements and may traverse several levels in their course into the subarachnoid space,

depending on the point at which the sinus was formed and how far the spinal cord ascended within the spinal canal from that point of development [20,21]. Patients who have dermal sinuses often have a skin dimple or a cutaneous pit in the midline of their back on physical examination. Other associated abnormalities include a tethered cord, (lipo) myelomeningocele, and vertebral body anomalies [15,20,21]. The tracts can be seen on cross-sectional imaging studies, such as MR imaging or sonography [20,21]. MR imaging may be helpful because it allows for visualization of the entire course of the sinus tract and the associated pathology(eg, skeletal abnormalities, spinal cord abnormalities such as syringohydromyelia, and masses such as dermoids and epidermoids) [15]. The sinus tract may enhance if infected, and abscess may occur along its tract.

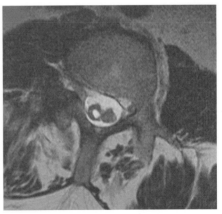

Fig. 14. Axial T2-weighted image shows two hemicords without intervening bar (type 2 diastematomyelia). The right hemicord contains a syrinx.

Spinal dermoid and epidermoid cysts (or nodules) are thought to develop secondary to ectodermal tissue remaining within the neural tube after primary neurulation [20,23,24]. These lesions are often associated with dermal sinus tracts but may also be found in isolation [20,22]. Histologically, epidermoid cysts have an outer wall of stratified squamous epithelium surrounded by a collagenous layer and a central cystic component created by desquamation and keratin breakdown, which may contain cholesterol crystals and fatty acids. Calcium may be present in the wall or within the cavity [23]. Dermoid cysts are similar but also contain skin appendages (ie, glandular elements and hair follicles) [25]. Both may be found in extradural, subdural, or intramedullary locations [23]. Epidermoid cysts are found most commonly in the thoracic spine between the levels of T5 and T8 [23]. Dermoid cysts are most commonly located in the lumbosacral spine but have also been reported in the cervical and thoracic spine [22,26]. Both may be seen in patients who have the Klippel-Feil syndrome. The findings on MR imaging are somewhat variable for dermoids and epidermoids. Homogeneous hypointense T1 and hyperintense T2 signals are typically seen, but heterogeneous signal intensity with patchy areas of enhancement has also been reported (Fig. 15A) [23]. Enhancement generally indicates current or previous infection. Diffusion-weighted imaging has been shown to be useful in the diagnosis of spinal epidermoid cysts, showing restricted diffusion within the lesion and thus allowing differentiation from other cystic masses (Fig. 15B) [27,28].

Spinal hamartomas are benign abnormally located rests of well differentiated mature ectodermal and mesodermal elements [23,29]. Their etiology is not known, but it has been postulated that it may be similar to intraspinal lipomas, where dorsal mesenchyme is able to enter the neural tube secondary to premature disjunction and is subsequently induced to form these hamartomatous elements by the neural tube [24]. Spinal hamartomas may be located in the cervical, thoracic, or lumbar spine and in the sacrum [23,29]. A true hamartoma of the spine or of the spinal cord contains only local elements (eg, nerves, blood vessels, fat, bone, cartilage, or synovial membranes), but other elements foreign to this location (eg, lymphoid tissue, glandular tissue, and urinary tract tissues) may be present [24]. Patients who have spinal hamartomas may have no external abnormalities, but there may be a skin dimple or angioma in the overlying skin or a subcutaneous mass. The masses are usually isointense to the spinal cord on T1- and T2-weighted MR imaging, and there may be associated widening of the spinal canal [24,29]. Symptoms may be due to compression of the spinal cord by the mass.

When all three germ cell layers are represented in a mass, the resulting tumor is called a "teratoma" (also referred to as a "monster neoplasm") [30]. Sacrococcygeal teratomas are the most common congenital tumors, probably arising from totipotential cells of Henson's node [30,31]. They are often associated with other abnormalities, including anorectal and genital malformations, ventricular septal defect, hip dislocation, and vertebral anomalies, such as spina bifida and sacral agenesis (Fig. 16) [30,32]. Several classifications exist for these tumors. Histologically, they are classified as mature or immature and graded from 0 to 3, with the grade increasing with the amount of immature tissue found in the tumor. Grade 0tumors have only mature tissues, whereas Grade 3 tumors have large

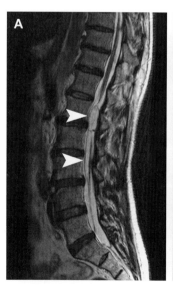
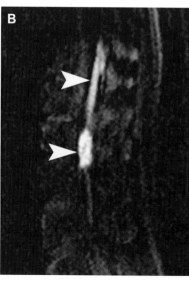

Fig. 15. (*A*) Sagittal T2-weighted image shows expansion of the filum terminale (*lower arrowhead*) and a mass (*upper arrowhead*) inferior to the conus medullaris. Both lesions were epidermoids. (*B*) In a different patient, sagittal diffusion–weighted image shows bright mass-like epidermoid (*lower arrowhead*), which extends superiorly (*upper arrowhead*) into the cord.

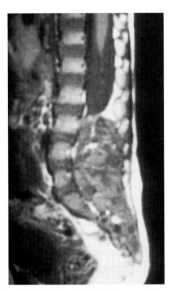

Fig. 16. Sagittal T1-weighted image shows partial sacral agenesis and a mostly intraspinal teratoma. Its inhomogenous signal intensities reflect its different tissue component. This teratoma does not fall into the typical classification proposed by the American Academy of Pediatrics.

amounts of immature tissue [30]. There is also a classification system used by the American Academy of Pediatrics' surgical section, which grades tumors by their anatomic extent (type I–IV). A type I tumor is mainly external, with a small presacral component; type II is characterized by external presentation with a large intrapelvic extension; type III is characterized by an external component with the majority of the tumor residing in the pelvis and abdomen; and type IV is entirely presacral, without an externally visible component [30,33]. Teratomas may be cystic, solid, or mixed, and more than 50% contain calcium [34]. These tumors are often first demonstrated on prenatal sonograms and are associated with polyhydramnios [34]. CT and MR imaging show a heterogeneous, enhancing mass with macroscopic fat; cystic areas and calcification are often seen. Although benign tumors are more likely to be predominantly cystic, imaging characteristics cannot reliably predict their histologic grade [34]. MR imaging is ideal for evaluating the intraspinal extension of these teratomas.

There is a spectrum of disorders that are seen when there is hypogenesis or agenesis of a portion of the spine, generally but not always in its distal aspects. Caudal regression syndrome (CRS) (also called "caudal agenesis syndrome") has been used to describe this phenomenon when it involves the most distal portions of the spine and sacrum and is associated with other congenital orthopedic,

cardiac, genitourinary, or gastrointestinal anomalies [10,35–37]. Some debate surrounds the pathogenesis of these lesions. Nievelstein and colleagues [35] suggest placing the patients into two groups: the first group having pathology best explained by an error in primary neurulation, with agenesis of parts of the spinal cord, nerve ganglia, and spine, and a second group, better explained by an error in the process of the degeneration and differentiation phase of development after normal primary and secondary neurulation, with vertebral agenesis and a tethered spinal cord that terminates at the level of the agenesis (Figs. 17 and 18). It has been suggested that this error may be related to the expression of the Hox gene, by a mutation or by a "loss-of-function" event, such as that created by environmental factors [36]. Over 30% of patients who have CRS are the offspring of diabetic mothers. Prenatal ultrasound examination in the second half of pregnancy may be limited by associated oligohydramnios, but lumbosacral agenesis may be discovered early in the second trimester [37]. Plain radiographs show hypoplasia or agenesis of osseous structures, but MR imaging is the mainstay of radiologic evaluation (Fig. 19) [10]. In the sagittal plane, there is often a characteristic wedge-shaped cord terminus, which is at times slightly longer on its dorsal aspect (see Fig. 18) [38]. The cord terminus in these cases is typically above the L1 level, but in situations where the spinal cord is tethered, it may terminate as low as the S2 level [10,35]. The cauda equina has a sparse appearance due to the

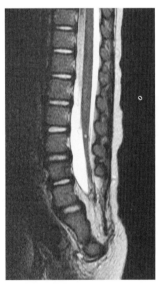

Fig. 17. Sagittal T2-weighted image shows partial sacral agenesis and a dysplastic cord that extends to the distal thecal sac and contains a tiny syrinx (type 2 caudal agenesis).

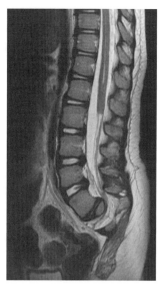

Fig. 18. Sagittal T2-weighted image in the more common type 1 sacral agenesis shows nearly complete absence of the sacrum and a conus medullaris that terminates bluntly. The cauda equina has a sparse appearance. The cord contains a syrinx.

lack of development of all of its nerve roots. Vertebral agenesis may begin in the thoracic spine in some cases but may begin as caudally as the S4 segment in others [35]. Sirenomyelia refers to the most severe manifestation of CRS. In these patients, the lower extremities are fused, the distal gastrointestinal and genitourinary tracts do not form normally, and the spine and cord may terminate as high as the

thoraco-lumbar region. Most of these cases are stillborn.

Segmental spinal dysgenesis refers to a similar process, but there is abnormal development of a segment (generally one vertebra) of the lumbar or thoracolumbar spine and respective spinal cord and/or nerve roots. There are vertebrae above and below the absent one, and often a bulky and low-lying segment of cord is found within the spinal canal caudally (Fig. 20) [39]. Plain radiographs of patients who have this rare condition show severe scoliosis or kyphoscoliosis and a variety of vertebral abnormalities. MR imaging not only shows the vertebral abnormalities; it is also useful in assessment of the spinal cord, which may be abnormally thin or indiscernible.

When scoliosis occurs congenitally, it is secondary to abnormal segmentation or formation of vertebral elements at one or multiple levels [40,41]. Examples of failure of formation are a wedge vertebra, where there is asymmetric height with relative hypoplasia of one chondrification center, and a hemivertebra, where one half of a vertebral body fails to form (Fig. 21). Hemivertebrae may be fully segmented, partially segmented, or unsegmented and are so called depending on the relative amounts of intervertebral disk space and fusion present at the levels above and below (hedequist). Occasionally associated with hemivertebrae are kyphotic (type A) or rotatory (type B), these deformities of the spinal column result in acute

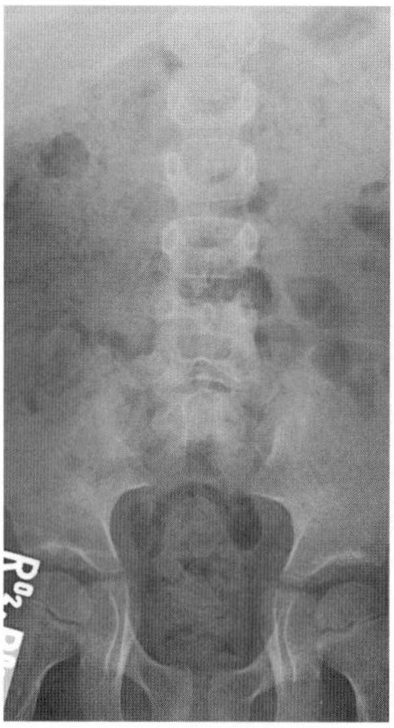

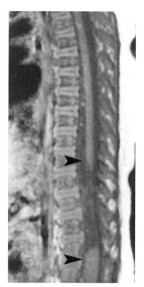

Fig. 20. Sagittal T1-weighted MR image shows the upper cord terminating abruptly (*upper arrowhead*) followed by a gap and then reappearance of a distal cord (*lower arrowhead*). This is a case of segmental spinal cord dysgenesis.

Fig. 19. Frontal radiograph shows complete agenesis of the sacrum.

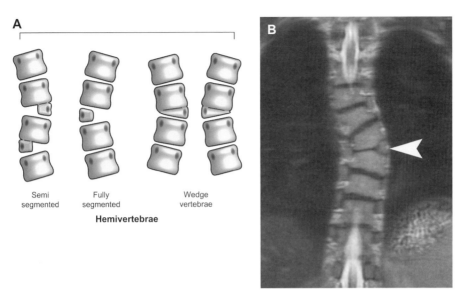

Fig. 21. (A) Different appearances and types of vertebral body fusions. (B) Coronal T2-weighted HASTE image shows levoscoliosis with a small remnant of a thoracic hemivertebra.

angulation, sometimes referred to as "congenital vertebral displacement" [42]. Segmentation defects may result in bony bars connecting two adjacent vertebrae (this is one of the most common identifiable causes of congenital scoliosis) (Fig. 22). When it occurs unilaterally, the result is a scoliosis, concave on the side of the bar. When it occurs bilaterally, there are block vertebrae (Fig. 23) [40]. The most severe scoliotic deformity is that seen when there is a combination of a segmentation defect with a contralateral formation defect [40]. The insult to the fetal spine causing congenital scoliosis

is thought to occur between the fifth and eighth weeks of gestation and may be related to mutations in genes that regulate segmentation and re-segmentation [41,43]. Congenital scoliosis is often associated with abnormalities in other organ systems, such as those seen in VACTERL syndrome (vertebral anomalies, anorectal atresia, cardiac defects, tracheoesophageal fistula, renal anomalies, and limb defects) [40]. Spinal dysraphism may be associated with congenital scoliosis [40]. Plain radiography is often used to classify the scoliotic deformity and to follow its progression over time, and

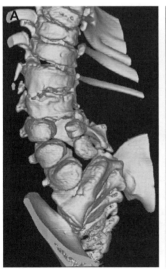
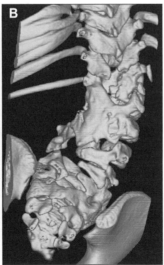

Fig. 22. (A) Anterior oblique three-dimensional CT view shows butterfly deformities at L3-L5, segmental fusion of L1 and L2, and scoliosis. (B) Same patient, posterior view. There is fusion of the posterior elements (right greater than left) of L1 and L2 due to an unsegmented posterior bar (Fig. 23A).

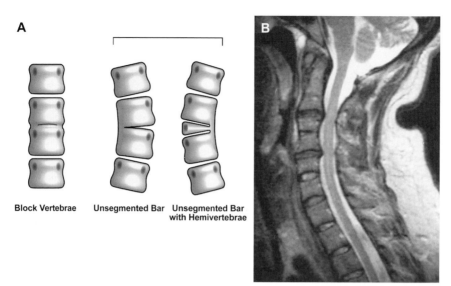

Fig. 23. (*A*) Diagram illustrating different types of vertebral fusions. (*B*) Sagittal T2-weighted MR image shows incidentally found fusion of C3 and C4. The fused vertebral bodies are smaller than the normal ones.

three-dimensional CT is used sometimes for defining the anatomy and for preoperative planning. MR imaging is also used for preoperative planning for assessment of a possible underlying intraspinal anomaly, which may be present in up to nearly 60% of these patients [40,44]. Spinal cord tethering, which is readily identified by MR imaging, is a contraindication to implantation of fixation devices.

Another rare entity that may result in scoliosis and/or kyphosis is the sagittal cleft vertebra or" butterfly vertebra." This results from failure of fusion of the two lateral chondrification centers of a vertebral body due to the persistent presence of the notochord within that vertebral segment [45,46]. Butterfly vertebrae usually occur in the lumbar or thoracic spine but have been reported in the cervical spine and occur more often in males [46,47]. The height of the affected segment is usually preserved when the hemivertebrae are bilateral and symmetric, but unilateral or bilateral hypoplasia may occur, resulting in scoliosis and/or kyphosis [46]. There may also be anterior wedging, which may be mistaken for a wedge fracture on a lateral radiograph, but the abnormality can be discerned in the anteroposterior view [45,46], which allows for identification of the typical butterfly shape. Butterfly vertebrae may be incidental but are often associated with syndromes such as Jarcho-Levin syndrome (spondylocostal/spondylothoracic dysostosis) or Alagille syndrome (paucity of interlobular bile ducts) [45,46,48]. Other spinal anomalies, such as diastematomyelia or spinal bifida, may accompany butterfly vertebrae [45].

The atlas may be hypoplastic, as in a hemi-atlas or hypoplasia of the posterior arch of the atlas, or partially or completely fused with the occiput [49]. Axis anomalies include odontoid hypo- or aplasia, where the basilar portion of the odontoid is partially or completely absent, and, rarely, congenital absence of the posterior elements of C2 (Fig. 24) [49–51]. One pedicle may be congenitally absent in rare instances. In and of itself this is a benign occurrence, but the radiographic findings (pseudo enlargement of the ipsilateral neural foramen, posterior displacement of the remaining ipsilateral posterior elements, or abnormal appearance

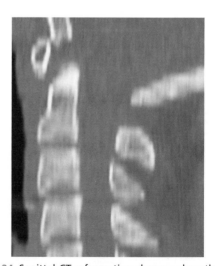

Fig. 24. Sagittal CT reformation shows a dens that is somewhat small and an anterior arch of C1 that is thick, elevated, and possibly fused with anterior border of the clivus. The posterior arch of C1 is not present.

of the ipsilateral transverse process) may mimic more serious pathology, such as acute trauma or a destructive or expanding lesion involving the pedicle and/or foramen; therefore, CT through the level of concern should be performed to make the diagnosis (Fig. 25) [52,53]. An os odontoideum is an ossicle that lies above the base of the odontoid. Once believed to be a congenital variant, it is more recently thought to be secondary to trauma [49]. The cervical spine may be studied with plain radiographs, often with additional lateral flexion and extension views to assess for translational instability. MR imaging also shows associated pathology, such as syringomyelia and compression of neural structure [49].

Patients who have a failure of segmentation in the cervical spine are grouped under the heading of Klippel-Feil syndrome [43]. Other abnormalities associated with Klippel-Feil syndrome include congenital scoliosis, Sprengel's deformity, deafness, cervical ribs and other rib abnormalities, and genitourinary and cardiac abnormalities [43]. Although the congenital spinal synostosis may occur at any level and involve multiple segments, it is most common at the C2-C3 level, followed by the C5-C6 level, with respective autosomal dominant and autosomal recessive inheritance patterns [49].

Summary

The complexity of the congenital anomalies of the spine can make the neuroradiologic diagnosis challenging. Knowledge of spinal embryology greatly helps in the understanding and classification of these anomalies. We have stressed the classification

devised by Tortori-Donati and Rossi [2], and we find it helpful from clinical and imaging standpoints. We believe that most patients who have known or suspected congenital spinal anomalies benefit from MR imaging.

References

[1] Rossi A, Biancheri R, Cama A, et al. Imaging in spine and spinal cord malformations. Eur J Radiol 2004;50:177–200.

[2] Tortori-Donati P, Rossi A, Cama A. Spinal dysraphism: a review of neuroradiological features with embryological correlations and proposal for a new classification. Neuroradiology 2000; 42:471–91.

[3] Guggisberg D, Hadj-Rabia S, Viney C, et al. Skin markers of occult spinal dysraphism. Arch Dermatol 2004;140:1109–15.

[4] Robinson AJ, Russell S, Rimmer S. The value of ultrasonic examination of the lumbar spine in infants with specific reference to cutaneous markers of occult spinal dysraphism. Clin Radiol 2005;60:72–7.

[5] Simon EM. MRI of the fetal spine. Pediatr Radiol 2004;34(9):712–9.

[6] Verity C, Firth H, French-Constant C. Congenital abnormalities of the central nervous system. J Neurol Neurosurg Psychiatry 2003;74:i3–8.

[7] Von Koch CS, Glenn OA, Goldstein RB, et al. Fetal magnetic resonance imaging enhances detection of spinal cord anomalies in patients with sonographically detected bony anomalies of the spine. J Ultrasound Med 2005;24:781–9.

[8] Sutton LN, Adzick NS. Fetal surgery for myelomeningocele. Clin Neurosurg 2004;51:155–62.

[9] Michelson DJ, Ashwal S. Tethered cord syndrome in childhood: diagnostic features and relationship to congenital anomalies. Neurol Res 2004; 26:745–53.

[10] Barkovich AJ. Pediatric neuroimaging, 3rd edition. Philadelphia: Lippincott Williams and Wilkins; 2000. p. 625–30, 650–3.

[11] Oner AY, Uzun M, Tokgoz N, et al. Isolated true anterior thoracic meningocele. AJNR Am J Neuroradiol 2004;25:1828–30.

[12] Massimi L, Calisti A, Koutzoglou M, et al. Giant anterior sacral meningocele and posterior sagittal approach. Childs Nerv Syst 2003;19:722–8.

[13] Unsinn KM, Geley T, Freund MC, et al. US of the spinal cord in newborns: spectrum of normal findings, variants, congenital anomalies, and acquired diseases. Radiographics 2000;20:923–38.

[14] Jesus LE, Franca CG. A rare variant of neuroenteric cyst: split notochord syndrome. J Pediatr (Rio J) 2004;80(1):77–80.

[15] Aydin K, Sencer S, Barman A, et al. Spinal cord herniation into a mediastinal neurenteric cyst: CT and MRI findings. Br J Radiol 2003;76:132–4.

[16] Rauzzino MJ, Tubbs RS, Alexander E, et al. Spinal neurenteric cysts and their relation to more

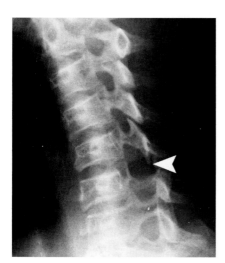

Fig. 25. Oblique radiograph of the cervical spine in a patient with pedicle agenesis shows a large C6-C7 neural foramen.

common aspects of occult spinal dysraphism. Neurosurg Focus 2001;10(1). Article 2.

[17] Kumar R, Jain R, Rao KM, et al. Intraspinal neurenteric cysts—report of three paediatric cases. Childs Nerv Syst 2001;17:584–8.

[18] Singhal BS, Parekh HN, Ursekar M, et al. Intramedullary neurenteric cyst in mid thoracic spine in an adult: a case report. Neurol India 2001;49: 302–4.

[19] Dias MS, Pang D. Split cord malformations. Neurosurg Clin N Am 1995;6(2):339–58.

[20] Kanev PM, Park TS. Dermoids and dermal sinus tracts of the spine. Neurosurg Clin N Am 1995;6: 359–66.

[21] Jindal A, Mahapatra AK. Spinal congenital dermal sinus: an experience of 23 cases over 7 years. Neurol India 2001;49:243–6.

[22] Shen WC, Chiou TL, Lin TY. Dermal sinus with dermoid cyst in the upper cervical spine: case note. Neuroradiology 2000;42:51–3.

[23] Lai SW, Chan WP, Chen C, et al. MRI of epidermoid cyst of the conus medullaris. Spinal Cord 2005;43:320–3.

[24] Castillo M, Smith MM, Armao D. Midline spinal cord hamartomas: MR imaging features of two patients. AJNR Am J Neuroradiol 1999;20: 1169–71.

[25] Castillo M. Neuroradiology: the core curriculum, 1st edition. Philadelphia: Lippincott Williams and Wilkins; 2002. p. 167.

[26] Sakai K, Sakamoto K, Kobayashi N, et al. Dermoid cyst within an upper thoracic meningocele. Surg Neurol 1996;45:287–92.

[27] Teksam M, Casey SO, Michel E, et al. Intraspinal epidermoid cyst: diffusion-weighted MRI. Neuroradiology 2001;43:572–4.

[28] Kikuchi K, Miki H, Nakagawa A. The utility of diffusion-weighted imaging with navigator-echo technique for the diagnosis of spinal epidermoid cysts. AJNR Am J Neuroradiol 2000; 21:1164–6.

[29] Morris GF, Murphy K, Rorke LB, et al. Spinal hamartomas: a distinct clinical entity. J Neurosurg 1998;88(6):954–7.

[30] Tuladhar R, Patole SK, Whitehall JS. Sacrococcygeal teratoma in the perinatal period. Postgrad Med J 2000;76:754–9.

[31] Wakhlu A, Misra S, Tandon RK, et al. Sacrococcygeal teratoma. Pediatr Surg Int 2002;18: 384–7.

[32] Lahdenne P, Heikinheimo M, Jaaskelainen J, et al. Vertebral abnormalities associated with congenital sacrococcygeal teratomas. J Pediatr Orthop 1991;11(5):603–7.

[33] Altman RP, Randolph JG, Lilly JR. Sacrococcygeal teratoma: American Academy of Pediatrics' surgical section survey—1973. J Pediatr Surg 1974;9: 389–98.

[34] Keslar PJ, Buck JL, Suarez ES. Germ cell tumors of the sacrococcygeal region: radiologic-pathologic correlation. Radiographics 1994;14:607–20.

[35] Nievelstein RAJ, Valk J, Smit LME, et al. MR of the caudal regression syndrome: embryologic implications. AJNR Am J Neuroradiol 1994;15:1021–9.

[36] Bohring A, Lewin SO, Reynolds JF, et al. Polytopic anomalies with agenesis of the lower vertebral column. Am J Med Genet 1999;87:99–114.

[37] Valenzano M, Paoletti R, Rossi A, et al. Pathological features, antenatal ultrasonographic clues, and a review of current embryogenic theories. Hum Reprod Update 1999;5:82–6.

[38] Barkovich AJ, Raghavan N, Chuang S, et al. The wedge-shaped cord terminus: a radiographic sign of caudal regression. AJNR Am J Neuroradiol 1989;10(6):1223–31.

[39] Tortori-Donati P, Fondelli MP, Rossi A, et al. Segmental spinal dysgenesis: neuroradiologic findings with clinical and embryologic correlation. AJNR Am J Neuroradiol 1999;20:445–56.

[40] Hedequist D, Emans J. Congenital scoliosis. J Am Acad Orthop Surg 2004;12:266–75.

[41] Arlet V, Odent T, Aebi M. Congenital scoliosis. Eur Spine J 2003;12:456–63.

[42] Shapiro J, Herring J. Congenital vertebral displacement. J Bone Joint Surg Am 1993;75: 656–62.

[43] Tracy MR, Dormans JP, Kusumi K. Klippel-Feil syndrome: clinical features and current understanding of etiology. Clin Orthop Relat Res 2004;424:183–90.

[44] Belmont PJ Jr, Kuklo TR, Taylor KF, et al. Intraspinal anomalies associated with isolated congenital hemivertebra: the role of routine magnetic resonance imaging. J Bone Joint Surg Am 2004; 86(8):1704–10.

[45] Sonel B, Yalcin P, Ozturk EA, et al. Butterfly vertebra: a case report. Journal of Clinical Imaging 2001;25:206–8.

[46] Brasili P, Bonfiglioli B, Ventrella AR. A case of butterfly vertebra from Sardinia. International Journal of Osteoarcheology 2002;12:415–9.

[47] Schlitt M, Dempsey PJ, Robinson RK. Cervical butterfly-block vertebra: a case report. Clin Imaging 1989;13(2):167–70.

[48] Teli M, Hosalkar H, Gill I, et al. Spondylocostal dysostosis. Spine 2004;29(13):1447–51.

[49] Guille JT, Sherk HH. Congenital osseous anomalies of the upper and lower cervical spine in children. J Bone Joint Surg Am 2002;84:277–88.

[50] Trivedi P, Vyas KH, Behari S. Congenital absence of the posterior elements of C2 vertebra: a case report. Neurol India 2003;51:250–1.

[51] Goel A, Gupta S, Laheri V. Congenital absence of posterior elements of axis: a report of two cases. Br J Neurosurg 1999;13(5):459–61.

[52] Gomez MA, Damie F, Besson M, et al. Congenital absence of a cervical spine pedicle: misdiagnosis in a context of trauma. Rev Chir Orthop Reparatrice Appar Mot 2003;89(8):738–41.

[53] Danziger J, Jackson H, Bloch S. Congenital absence of a pedicle in a cervical vertebra. Clin Radiol 1975;26(1):53–6.

**NEUROIMAGING
CLINICS
OF NORTH AMERICA**

Neuroimag Clin N Am 17 (2007) 17–35

ELSEVIER
SAUNDERS

Tumors of the Spine in Children

Andrea Rossi, MD*, Carlo Gandolfo, MD,
Giovanni Morana, MD, Paolo Tortori-Donati, MD

- Intramedullary tumors
  Astrocytoma
  Ganglioglioma
  Ependymoma
- Intradural-extramedullary tumors
  Myxopapillary ependymoma
  Nerve sheath tumors
  Meningioma
  Atypical teratoid rhabdoid tumor
  Primitive neuroectodermal tumors

- *Dysontogenetic and non-neoplastic
  masses*
- Extradural tumors
  *Benign bone tumors and tumor-like
  conditions*
  Malignant bone tumors
  Tumors of the epidural spaces
  *Extraspinal tumors with spinal
  invasion*
- References

In children, tumors of the spine are much rarer than intracranial tumors (approximately 1:10). They are classified into intramedullary, intradural-extramedullary, and extradural tumors. In our experience, extradural tumors account for about two thirds of cases, intramedullary tumors for one fourth, and intradural-extramedullary tumors for the remainder.

Because of an aspecific clinical presentation, most children are initially imaged with conventional x-rays. Intradural (intra- and extramedullary) tumors cause enlargement of the spinal canal and vertebral scalloping, but these signs are not early indicators of the underlying disease. Conversely, extradural tumors usually produce more evident involvement of bone already in the early stages. Magnetic resonance (MR) imaging provides crucial information regarding the extent, location, and internal structure of the mass, thus critically narrowing the differential diagnosis and guiding surgery [1,2]. The MR imaging technique ideally includes

the use of phased-array surface coils and must include unenhanced sagittal T1- and T2-weighted images and contrast-enhanced T1-weighted images in all three planes of space; axial T2-weighted images are used to detect spinal cord compression from extrinsic tumors. Computerized tomography (CT) plays an important role in the assessment of bone tumors and in detecting calcifications; spiral volumetric acquisitions improve the quality of multiplanar reformatting. The clinical role of advanced MR imaging modalities, including MR spectroscopy, diffusion-weighted imaging, diffusion tensor imaging, and functional MR imaging, has not been extensively researched.

Intramedullary tumors

Intramedullary tumors account for 4% to 10% of all primary central nervous system (CNS) neoplasms and for 25% of pediatric spinal tumors [1]. They prevail in children between 1 and 5 years of age

Department of Pediatric Neuroradiology, G. Gaslini Children's Hospital, Largo G. Gaslini 5, I-16147 Genoa, Italy
* Corresponding author.
E-mail address: andrearossi@ospedale-gaslini.ge.it (A. Rossi).

doi:10.1016/j.nic.2006.11.004
neuroimaging.theclinics.com

without gender prevalence. Astrocytomas are the most common intramedullary tumor in the pediatric age group (82% of cases) [1], followed by gangliogliomas. Ependymomas are uncommon in children outside the setting of neurofibromatosis Type 2.

The presentation, duration, and course of the disease may be variable. Affected patients may have a prolonged duration of symptoms before a diagnosis is established. Symptoms may be elicited by trauma or efforts. Back pain is often the earliest and most persistent complaint and should prompt to MR imaging to rule out intraspinal pathology. Rigidity and contracture of the paravertebral muscles may result from thecal sac enlargement, involvement of adjacent bone, and impaired of cerebrospinal fluid (CSF) dynamics. Progressive scoliosis may cause delays in the diagnosis if underestimated. Head tilt and torticollis and lower cranial nerve palsies with dysphagia, dyspnea, and dysphonia may represent early signs of cervico-medullary neoplasms due to involvement of the spinal roots of the accessory nerve innervating the trapezius and sternocleidomastoid muscles. Sensorimotor disturbances generally occur later in the course of disease and may be difficult to evaluate, especially in small children. Long-lasting weakness and spinal or limb muscle atrophy may be found with slowly growing tumors [3,4]. Hydrocephalus with raised intracranial pressure may rarely represent the clinical presentation of intramedullary tumors and is caused by obstruction of the spinal subarachnoid spaces, CSF seeding, or increased CSF protein content [5].

On MR imaging, intramedullary neoplasms produce enlargement of the spinal cord, giving heterogeneous signal intensity. They may be solid or associated with neoplastic or non-neoplastic cysts. Neoplastic cysts are located within the tumor mass, result from necrosis and degeneration, show peripheral enhancement on gadolinium-enhanced sequences, and must be removed surgically. Non-neoplastic cysts are located at the cranial and caudal poles of the tumor, result from reactive dilatation of the central canal due to tumor fluid secretion or mechanical blockage of the ependymal canal, have unenhancing margins, and can be drained and aspirated but not resected [6]. Swelling of the spinal cord cranial and caudad to the tumor can result from edema. Discrimination of tumor from nonneoplastic areas such as polar cysts and edema is crucial for surgical planning.

Astrocytoma

In the pediatric age group, astrocytomas account for the vast majority of intrinsic spinal cord neoplasms, with most tumors being low grade (ie, pilocytic and fibrillary) [2,7]. In our experience, pilocytic astrocytomas account for 75% of all intramedullary tumors in the pediatric age group and typically affect children between 1 and 5 years of age, whereas fibrillary astrocytomas account for 7% and tend to occur in older children (around 10 years of age) [1].

On MR imaging, pilocytic astrocytomas are characterized by enlargement of the spinal cord within a widened spinal canal. They frequently involve a large portion of the cord, spanning multiple vertebral levels in length. True "holocord" tumors are rare; in most cases, involvement of the whole length of the spinal cord is caused by extensive spinal cord edema rather than by a tumor. The cervico-medullary junction and the cervico-thoracic cord are the most common locations. Tumors can show areas of necrotic-cystic degeneration (60% of cases), can have a "cyst with mural nodule" appearance (Fig. 1), or can be structurally solid (about 40% of cases) (Fig. 2). The solid components are iso- to hypointense on T1-weighted images and hyperintense on T2-weighted images, whereas necrotic-cystic components display higher relaxation times on T1- and T2-weighted images. Some degree of contrast enhancement is present in the majority of spinal cord pilocytic astrocytomas. The pattern of enhancement is variable and does not define tumor margins [1].

Ganglioglioma

Gangliogliomas are the second most common intramedullary tumor in the pediatric age group (15% of cases) and mostly affect children between 1 and 5 years of age, as do pilocytic astrocytomas [1] Although they typically are low-grade tumors (Grade I-II) with a low potential for malignant degeneration, they have a significant propensity for local recurrence [8], and the glial element may progress to high grade. Their preferential location is in the cervical and upper thoracic cord with extension to the medulla through the foramen magnum. Holocord involvement has been described to be more frequent than in other spinal cord tumors, probably as a result of low growth rate [9], but we have not had similar results [1]. Although propensity for cyst formation has been reported to be common [2], all gangliogliomas in our series were predominantly solid [1].

On imaging, calcification is probably the single most suggestive feature of gangliogliomas (Fig. 3) [1]. In the absence of gross calcification, the MR imaging appearance of gangliogliomas is nonspecific and does not allow differentiation from astrocytomas. Solid portions have mixed iso-hypointensity on T1-weighted images and heterogeneous iso-hyperintensity on T2-weighted images [10]. Perifocal

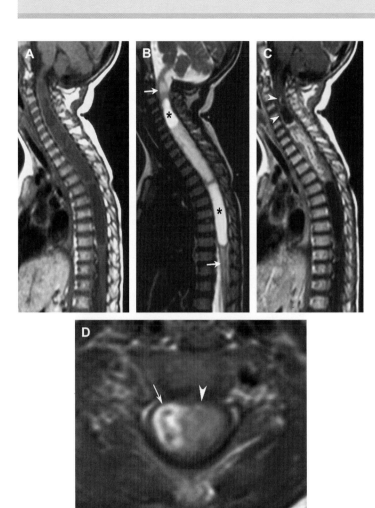

Fig. 1. Pilocytic astrocytoma in an 18-month-old boy. (*A*) Sagittal T1-weighted and (*B*) sagittal T2-weighted image show large tumor with a solid component extending from C6 to T5 and two large peripheral cysts (*asterisks*). The solid component is hypointense on T1-weighted images and hyperintense on T2-weighted images. There is cord edema above and below the tumor (*arrows*). (*C*) Gadolinium-enhanced, sagittal T1-weighted image shows the solid portion of the tumor enhances strongly and inhomogeneously. Enhancement of the walls of the cranial cyst indicates a neoplastic cyst (*arrowheads*). (*D*) Gadolinium-enhanced, axial T1-weighted MR image shows inhomogeneously enhancing lesion due to mixed necrotic (*arrow*) and solid (*arrowhead*) components.

edema can vary from limited or absent [10] to extensive (Fig. 4). Contrast enhancement can be focal or patchy, and it rarely involves the whole tumor mass; absence of enhancement has also been described in a minority of cases [11].

Ependymoma

Spinal cord ependymomas are virtually nonexistent in the pediatric age group outside the setting of neurofibromatosis Type 2. While they may extend over large portions of the cord, most neurofibromatosis Type 2–related ependymomas are small intramedullary nodules that may be multiple. These markedly vascularized tumors frequently show intralesional hemorrhages, which constitute their hallmark also on neuroimaging, producing the so-called "cap sign," a T2 hypointense rim surrounding the cranial or caudal poles of the lesion that results from magnetic susceptibility effects [12].

Intradural-extramedullary tumors

In the pediatric age group, most intradural-extramedullary tumors are leptomeningeal metastases from primary brain tumors. Primitive tumors in this location are the least common among spinal tumors and are mostly represented by schwannomas and neurofibromas in neurofibromatosis patients. A host of other neoplasms, including filar ependymomas, meningiomas, and atypical teratoid rhabdoid tumors, can be found in this location. Other lesions include dysontogenetic masses and other non-neoplastic masses. Clinical features are represented by pain and signs of cord or nerve root compression, depending on the location of the mass. Only primitive intradural-extramedullary tumors are discussed in this article.

Myxopapillary ependymoma

Myxopapillary ependymomas account for 13% of all spinal ependymomas in the general population;

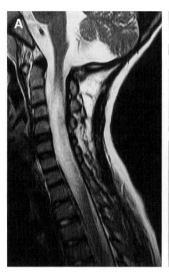
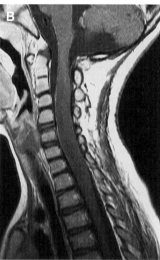

Fig. 2. Pilocytic astrocytoma in a 2-year-old girl. (*A*) Sagittal T2-weighted MR image shows ill-defined hyperintense lesion expanding the cervical spinal cord. (*B*) Gadolinium-enhanced, sagittal T1-weighted MR image shows absence of enhancement.

however, they are more frequent in the pediatric age group. They are thought to arise from the ependymal glia of the filum terminale and typically present as intradural extramedullary lesions involving the lumbar and sacral canal [13]. Rarely, myxopapillary ependymomas involve the sacrococcygeal region, arising from vestiges at the distal portion of the neural tube [14]. Affected patients present with lower back, leg, or sacral pain; weakness or sphincter dysfunction [2]; and occasionally subarachnoid hemorrhage [6].

On MR imaging, the lesion is iso- to hyperintense on T1-weighted images and hyperintense on T2-weighted images. Contrast enhancement is moderate to marked and may be inhomogeneous. It is not uncommon for large masses to envelope or infiltrate the outer surface of the conus medullaris (Fig. 5). Large masses may extend into the neural foramina, expand the spinal canal, and erode the adjacent vertebrae [13]. The main differential diagnosis is with nerve sheath tumors, such as schwannomas.

Nerve sheath tumors

Schwannomas

Schwannomas, or neurinomas, originate from Schwann cells in the sheaths of spinal root and nerves and grow extrinsically with respect to the axon. They are separated from the adjacent tissues

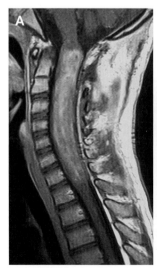
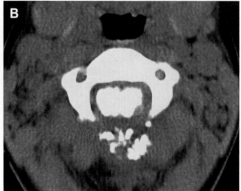

Fig. 3. Ganglioglioma in a 7-year-old boy. (*A*) Gadolinium-enhanced, sagittal T1-weighted MR image shows cervical intramedullary tumor causing expansion of the spinal canal. This mass was spontaneously hyperintense on unenhanced T1-weighted images (not shown). (*B*) Axial CT scan obtained after laminectomy shows a coarsely calcified intramedullary mass.

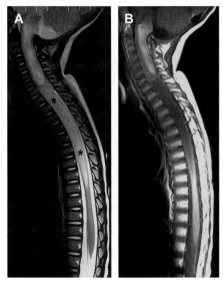

Fig. 4. Ganglioglioma in a 10-month-old boy. (A) Sagittal T2-weighted MR image shows hyperintense cervical intramedullary tumor with extensive spinal cord edema (*asterisks*). (B) Gadolinium-enhanced, sagittal T1-weighted MR image shows enhancement of the tumor, clearly demarcating it from the associated edema.

by a thin capsule, which facilitates surgical removal. Isolated spinal schwannomas are rare in the pediatric population, whereas multiple schwannomas in the setting of neurofibromatosis Type 2 are more frequent. They may be intradural, extradural, or both, depending on where they originate along the course of the spinal root; however, intradural tumors are more common. Within the lumbar thecal sac, they may attain a considerable size before

becoming clinically manifest, causing enlargement of the spinal canal, scalloping, and bone erosion. On MR imaging, schwannomas are iso- to hypointense on T1-weighted images and iso- to hyperintense in T2-weighted images. Contrast enhancement is moderate to marked and essentially homogeneous (Fig. 6).

Neurofibromas

Neurofibromas are composed of an admixture of Schwann cells and fibroblasts and tend to infiltrate, rather than dislocate, the root or nerve from which they originate. Therefore, radical surgery is usually much more difficult to attain than with schwannomas. Neurofibromas are typically found in patients with neurofibromatosis type 1. They may be solitary or multiple (Fig. 7) and may resemble a string of beads when they affect multiple nerve roots in the thecal sac. On MR imaging, their behavior is similar to that of schwannomas, with iso- to hypointensity on T1-weighted images, hyperintensity on T2-weighted images, and marked contrast enhancement.

Meningioma

Meningiomas are uncommon tumors in the pediatric age group outside the setting of neurofibromatosis type 2. Isolated spinal meningiomas typically belong to a particular histologic variant called "clear cell meningioma." Clear cell meningiomas are typical of younger patients, are prevailingly located in the spinal canal and cerebellopontine angle, and show a more aggressive behavior with higher recurrence rate and propensity for leptomeningeal dissemination than adult subtypes [15–18].

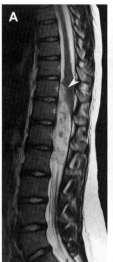
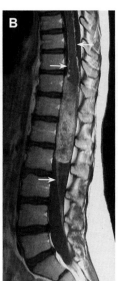
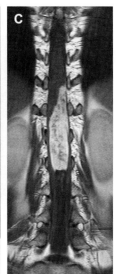

Fig. 5. Myxopapillary ependymoma in a 10-year-old boy. (A) Sagittal T2-weighted MR image and (B) gadolinium-enhanced, sagittal T1-weighted MR image show intradural-extradural thoracolumbar mass that infiltrated the outer surface of the cord (*arrowhead*, A). There is venous congestion over the surface of the cord and in the caudal thecal sac (*arrows*, B). (C) Gadolinium-enhanced, coronal T1-weighted MR image shows slightly inhomogeneous tumor enhancement.

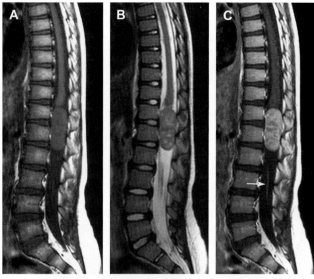

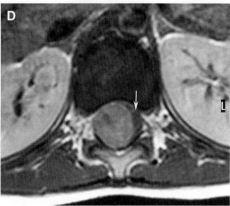

Fig. 6. Schwannoma in a 5-year-old girl. (A) Sagittal T1-weighted MR image shows smoothly marginated intradural-extramedullary mass that is essentially isointense with the spinal cord. (B) On sagittal T2-weighted MR image the lesion is mildly hyperintense and contains a few higher-intensity spots. (C) Gadolinium-enhanced, sagittal T1-weighted MR image shows moderate, slightly inhomogeneous tumor enhancement and venous congestion in the thecal sac caudad to the lesion (arrow). (D) Gadolinium-enhanced, axial T1-weighted MR image shows marked displacement of the apex of the conus medullaris (arrow) by this large intradural-extramedullary mass.

On MR imaging, clear cell meningiomas are round to ovoid, well demarcated masses that are isointense to the spinal cord on T1- and T2-weighted images. Contrast enhancement is moderate to marked and homogeneous (Fig. 8). As with conventional meningiomas, the presence of a dural tail sign is not mandatory [17].

Atypical teratoid rhabdoid tumor

Atypical teratoid rhabdoid tumors (ATRT) are highly malignant neoplasms that are ubiquitous in the CNS. Although most affect the brain, they may primitively involve the spine [19]. Owing to their marked aggressiveness, primitively extra-axial lesions may infiltrate the spinal cord and vice versa, so that the origin of the tumor may be difficult to assess on neuroimaging. ATRTs predominate in the first 2 years of life and may be congenital.

Neuroimaging features (Fig. 9) are similar to those of intracranial ATRTs [20]. These tumors are structurally heterogeneous due to often extensive

hemorrhage and necrotic-cystic change. Solid portions are hypointense on T1- and T2-weighted images due to marked cellularity with high nuclear-to-cytoplasmatic ratio. Contrast enhancement is inhomogenous. MR imaging of the whole neuraxis must be performed to identify possible secondary spread or multicentric disease.

Primitive neuroectodermal tumors

Primitive neuroectodermal tumors (PNETs) are composed by undifferentiated or poorly differentiated cells and belong to a category of infantile, aggressive neoplasms, including neuroblastomas and Ewing sarcomas, which are characterized histologically by a monotonous hypercellularity composed by small, round cells with hyperchromatic nucleus and scant cytoplasm [21]. Intraspinal PNETs are rare and more often occur in older children than in intracranial PNETs [22–24].

Neuroimaging features of intraspinal PNETs are nonspecific. Our experience is that of a single case

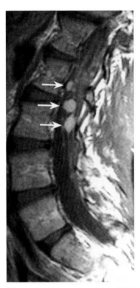

Fig. 7. Neurofibromas in a 12-year-old boy with neurofibromatosis Type 1. Gadolinium-enhanced, sagittal T1-weighted MR image shows bunch of neurofibromas of the cauda equina appearing as markedly enhancing, multiple nodular masses (*arrows*).

originating from an intradural-extramedullary location in the cervical spine and causing spinal compression (Fig. 10). This lesion was isointense with the spinal cord on T1- and T2-weighted images and enhanced homogeneously.

Dysontogenetic and non-neoplastic masses

(Epi)dermoids

Dermoids account for 10% of all spinal tumors in the pediatric age group and are often associated with dermal sinuses [25]; they may be primitive or iatrogenic (ie, secondary to inadvertent inclusion of skin debris during surgical interventions, such as myelomeningocele repair). Epidermoids are relatively infrequent in the pediatric age group.

Structurally, dermoids have a cystic structure lined by squamous epithelium containing dermal appendages (eg, hair, sweat glands, and sebaceous glands), whereas epidermoids are lined by squamous epithelium lacking cutaneous appendages. The fluid within both lesions contains cutaneous debris with variable concentrations of keratin, whose accumulation causes them to enlarge slowly. Complications include abscess formation and rupture of the cyst into the subarachnoid spaces, causing chemical meningitis.

(Epi)dermoids may be difficult to identify on conventional MR imaging because their signal intensity is similar to that of CSF (Fig. 11). Proton-density and fluid attenuated inversion recovery (FLAIR) sequences are usually more sensitive than T1- or T2-weighted images. Diffusion-weighted imaging is useful, showing restricted diffusion within the cyst. Contrast enhancement is usually absent, except in case of superinfection.

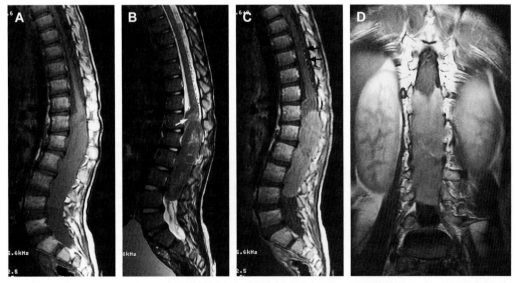

Fig. 8. Clear cell meningioma in a 5-year-old girl. Sagittal T1-weighted MR image (*A*), sagittal T2-weighted MR image (*B*), and gadolinium-enhanced, sagittal T1-weighted MR image (*C*) show huge intradural lesion extending from T12 to L4, characterized by isointensity with cord on T1-weighted (*A*) and T2-weighted images (*B*). There is moderate enhancement after gadolinium administration (*C*). The spinal canal is enlarged. The conus medullaris is deformed and compressed and shows signal changes consistent with edema (*arrow, B*). There is venous congestion over the ventral and dorsal surface of the spinal cord (*arrows, C*). (*D*) Gadolinium-enhanced, coronal T1-weighted MR image confirms huge lesion expanding the thecal sac.

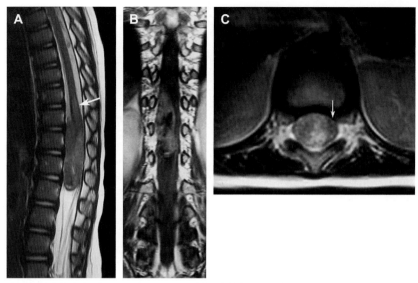

Fig. 9. Atypical teratoid rhabdoid tumor in a 2-year-old girl. (*A*) Sagittal T2-weighted MR image shows huge iso- to hyperintense lesion extending from T11 to L2, causing spinal cord edema (*arrow*). (*B*) Gadolinium-enhanced, coronal T1-weighted MR image shows that enhancement is marked and inhomogeneous. (*C*) Axial T2-weighted MR image shows that the mass is intradurally located and markedly compresses and displaces the conus medullaris to the left (*arrow*). At surgery, the lesion was found to originate from the right T12 nerve root.

Neurenteric cysts

Neurenteric cysts have a congenital origin from remnants of the primitive streak during early embryonic development. They are lined with a mucin-secreting, cuboidal or columnar epithelium that resembles the alimentary tract [25]. Their content is variable, and the chemical composition may be similar to CSF, which is reflected into a variable pattern of signal intensity on MR imaging. They are more frequently located in the cervicothoracic spine anterior to the cord.

Arachnoid cysts

Arachnoid cysts are CSF collections housed within a splitting of the arachnoid membrane that do not communicate with the subarachnoid space. In the spine, arachnoid cysts may be located in the subdural or, less often, in the epidural space dorsal to the cord. They may be congenital or may result from adhesions provoked by previous infection or trauma. As such, they may complicate surgery for spinal dysraphism and may cause subsequent neurologic deterioration with signs of cord tethering.

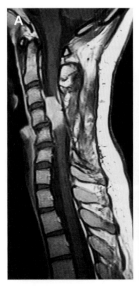

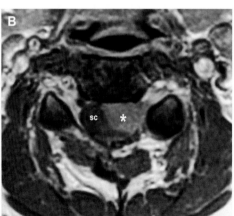

Fig. 10. Primitive neuroectodermal tumor in a 17-year-old girl. (*A*) Gadolinium-enhanced, sagittal T1-weighted MR image shows intradural-extramedullary mass in the cervical spine at the C4 level. (*B*) Gadolinium-enhanced axial T1-weighted MR image shows that the mass (*asterisk*) causes contralateral displacement of the spinal cord (sc). After 8 months, a metastatic nodule was discovered in the distal thecal sac (not shown).

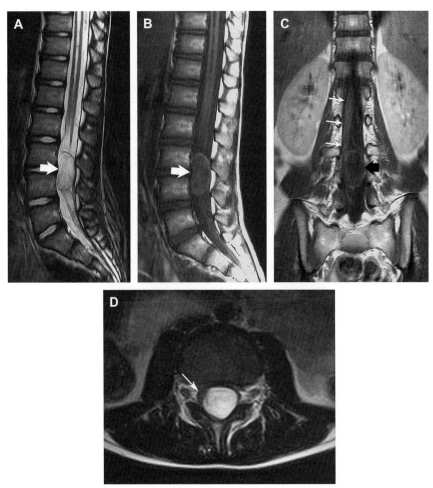

Fig. 11. Dermoid in a 6-year-old boy. Sagittal T1-weighted (*A*) and T2-weighted (*B*) MR images show smoothly marginated intradural lesion at L3-4 (*arrow*). The mass gives similar signal intensity to CSF in both sequences. There is concurrent hydromyelia. (*C*) Gadolinium-enhanced, coronal T1-weighted MR image shows the lesion is not enhancing (*black arrow*). There is displacement of the conus medullaris (*thin arrows*). (*D*) Axial T2-weighted MR image shows relationship between the intradural mass at L3 and the displaced conus tip (*arrow*).

On MR imaging, the signal intensity of arachnoid cysts parallels that of CSF in all sequences. Some arachnoid cysts may contain proteinaceous fluid or blood, thereby resulting in increased T1 and T2 relaxation times, which may pose diagnostic problems. They may cause enlargement of the spinal canal and mild compression of the posterior aspect of the cord. Cine-MR imaging is useful to demonstrate exclusion of the cyst from the surrounding subarachnoid spaces and to monitor surgical results.

Extradural tumors

Extradural tumors account for about two thirds of all spinal tumors in the pediatric age group and may be grouped into bone tumors, tumors of the

epidural space, and extraspinal tumors invading the spine. Affected children usually complain of back pain and myeloradiculopathy. Neuroimaging of extradural tumors requires MR imaging and CT. MR imaging depicts extradural soft tissue components, bone marrow infiltration, and myelopathy due to extrinsic compression from the tumor, whereas CT detects the osteolytic or osteosclerotic nature of the lesion and the degree of involvement of bone.

Benign bone tumors and tumor-like conditions

Hemangioma

Vertebral hemangiomas are usually discovered incidentally. They involve the vertebral body and may be solitary or multiple. They are composed of capillary and cavernous spaces, lined by endothelium and surrounded by adipose tissue and thickened, sclerotic trabeculae that have a compensatory function. In some instances, lymphatic components are present. Although most vertebral hemangiomas are dormant lesions, some show an aggressive behavior with expansion of involved bone, epidural extension, and vertebral collapse, in which case patients experience local pain and may develop signs of spinal cord and nerve root compression.

On radiograph and CT, vertebral hemangiomas produce a palisading appearance of vertical sclerotic densities in the vertebral body. On MR imaging, end-stage, dormant angiomas are hyperintense on T1- and T2-weighted images due to fatty and vascular components, and the affected vertebra is morphologically normal. Instead, potentially aggressive hemangiomas are low intensity on T1-weighted images, bright on T2-weighted images, and cause bone expansion, resulting in a swollen appearance of the affected bone (Fig. 12).

Osteoid osteoma

Approximately 10% of all osteoid osteomas are located in the spine, usually involving the posterior vertebral elements. Affected patients usually present with nocturnal pain, which recedes with nonsteroid anti-inflammatory medications, or with painful scoliosis. Histologically, the tumor is composed of a richly vascularized nidus of osteoid bone containing a sclerotic center, surrounded by marked reactive osteosclerosis. Reactive inflammatory soft-tissue masses often surround the bony lesion and may extensively involve the paravertebral regions [26,27].

Radionuclide bone scans are extremely sensitive in the detection of osteoid osteomas (Fig. 13). CT shows the nidus as a rounded hypodense lesion surrounded by a hyperdense sclerotic ring. Calcification within the nidus results in a target appearance of the lesion (see Fig. 13). On MR imaging, the nidus is hyperintense on T2-weighted images and enhances markedly; the surrounding osteosclerotic component results in a hypointense ring. Because of the small size of the lesion, accuracy of MR imaging in identification of osteoid osteomas is not high (65%) [28]. MR imaging clearly detects the extensive reactive soft-tissue masses that are frequently associated with the osteoma (see Fig. 13). In one study, gadolinium-enhanced MR imaging was not inferior to thin-section CT in the detection of osteoid osteomas [29].

Osteoblastoma

It is classically believed that osteoblastomas differ from osteoid osteomas only in size (>2 cm in diameter) [30]. Although the two tumors are indistinguishable histologically, osteoblastomas often show an aggressive behavior, with huge infiltrating masses that may bleed extensively during surgery. There is a predilection for the neural arch, as with osteoid osteomas, but the lesion may extend into the vertebral body and paraspinal soft tissues. Patients present with aspecific pain that does not recede with salicylates.

In typical cases, CT shows an expansile lytic lesion, possibly associated with sclerotic components. Although osteoblastomas are histologically benign, they may show atypical features that mimic more aggressive lesions, including bone destruction,

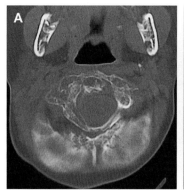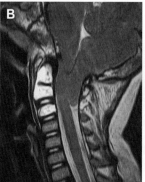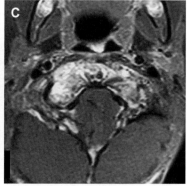

Fig. 12. Cystic angiomatosis of the craniovertebral junction in a 5-year-old boy. (*A*) Axial CT scan shows diffuse lytic process involving the odontoid process of C2, the atlas, the posterior margin of the foramen magnum, and the occiput. The affected bone is slightly expanded. (*B*) Sagittal T2-weighted image shows diffuse signal abnormality involving the clivus, occipital squama, and C1 to C3. There is discrete swelling of C2 and concurrent downward ectopia of the cerebellar tonsils consistent with a Chiari I malformation. (*C*) Gadolinium-enhanced, fat-suppressed axial T1-weighted image shows intense contrast enhancement of the affected bone.

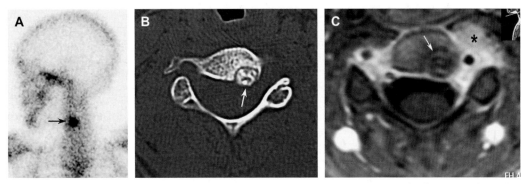

Fig. 13. Osteoid osteoma in an 8-year-old girl. (A) Radionuclide bone scan shows markedly increased uptake at C4 (*arrow*). (B) Axial CT scan shows the typical appearance of an osteoid osteoma (ie, a target lesion characterized by central sclerosis and surrounding radiolucency) (*arrow*). Somewhat atypically, this lesion involves the vertebral body instead of the neural arch. (C) Gadolinium-enhanced, axial T1-weighted image confirms the target appearance of the lesion (*arrow*) and shows enhancing reactive soft tissue mass in the homolateral neural foramen and paravertebral region (*asterisk*).

hemorrhage, and soft tissue components with resulting thecal sac and cord compression (Fig. 14). On MR imaging, signal intensity is heterogeneous on T1- and T2-weighted images. Gadolinium enhancement is marked, and vascularity may be prominent.

Aneurysmal bone cysts

Aneurysmal bone cysts (ABCs) probably are not neoplasms; rather, they may be reactive lesions that may result from trauma or coexist with other benign or malignant bone lesions [31,32]. In our experience, ABCs have accounted for 42% of all benign bone tumors in children [1]. About 75% are located in the lower thoracic and lumbosacral spine, whereas the remainder involve the cervical spine. They usually originate from the neural arch but may extend to the body along one, or rarely both, vertebral pedicles and may cross disk spaces to involve adjacent vertebral levels [31,32]. These osteolytic lesions have a multicystic structure composed of wide, communicating

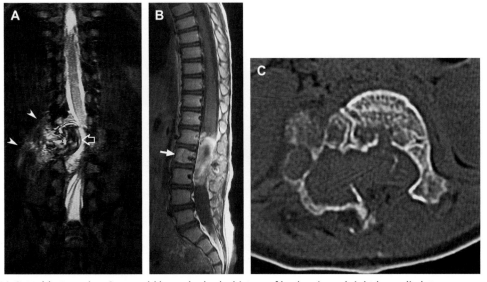

Fig. 14. Osteoblastoma in a 2-year-old boy who had a history of back pain and right lower limb tremor progressing to paresis and then inability to walk within 2 days. (A) Coronal T2-weighted short time inversion recovery MR image shows a huge soft tissue mass that involves extensively the intraspinal compartment and the paravertebral regions to the right (*arrowheads*). The intraspinal portion is hemorrhagic (*open arrow*). (B) Gadolinium-enhanced, sagittal T1-weighted MR image shows extensive intraspinal component at L1-3 and partial L2 vertebral body collapse (*arrow*). (C) Axial CT scan at L2 shows extensive osteolysis with disruption of the right peduncle.

loculations that contain unclotted blood separated by thin calcified shells. Affected patients usually are older children or adolescents complaining of local pain, possibly associated with myelopathy or radiculopathy [1].

On neuroimaging (Fig. 15), ABCs are osteolytic, expansile, sometimes destructive lesions. On CT, the lesion is composed of multiple cystic spaces separated by thin, calcified shells. On MR imaging, signal intensity is variable depending on the blood degradation by-products contained within the cysts [31,32]. Multiple dependent intralesional fluid–fluid levels are typically found and constitute the hallmark of ABCs (see Fig. 15). Fluid–fluid levels may also be found in other tumors, including giant cell tumors and telangiectatic osteosarcomas [33], which, however, are exceptionally found in

children. Due to their hypervascularity, ABCs may be amenable to presurgical embolization to reduce intraoperative bleeding [34].

Eosinophilic granulomas

Langerhans cell histiocytosis is a reactive disorder of unknown etiology ranging from a multisystem disease (Letterer-Siwe and Hand-Schuller-Christian diseases) to a single-system disease confined to the skeleton (eosinophilic granuloma) [35]. Eosinophilic granulomas of the spine affect the vertebral body and typically result in somatic collapse. As the end plates remain intact, the adjacent disks are consistently unaffected and may show compensatory swelling. Preservation of the growth plates allows for subsequent reconstitution of vertebral height, which may be more efficient in younger patients

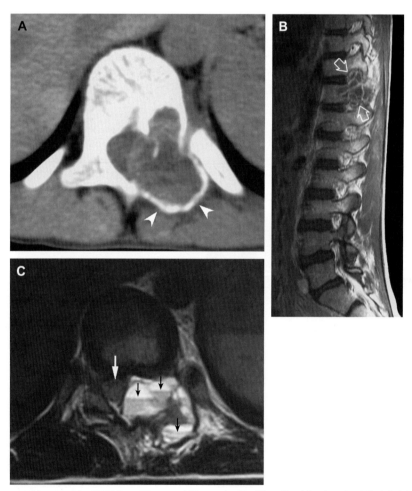

Fig. 15. Aneurysmal bone cyst of T11 in a 12-year-old boy who had localized back pain. (*A*) Axial CT scan shows lytic expansile lesion of the posterior neural arch of T11 to the left, delimited by a thin calcified shell (*arrowheads*). (*B*) Gadolinium-enhanced, sagittal T1-weighted MR image shows multiloculated mass with enhancing septations that replaces the left peduncle of T11 (*arrows*). (*C*) Axial T2-weighted MR image shows multiple dependent fluid–fluid levels (*thin arrows*). The spinal cord, albeit displaced, does not show signal abnormalities (*thick arrow*), which is consistent with the normal neurologic picture.

[36]. Involvement of the posterior elements of the spine is exceptional [37]. Patients present with pain and general symptoms, including fever and weight loss. The cervical spine is involved in as many as three fourths of cases [1].

Radiographs and CT with multiplanar reconstructions typically show an osteolytic lesion causing a variable degree of vertebral collapse. MR imaging also shows vertebral collapse with compensatory swelling of the adjacent disks. The pathologic vertebra enhances markedly and often is associated with enhancing soft tissue components that may involve the anterior epidural space and compress the thecal sac (Fig. 16). Other causes of vertebral collapse in children include lymphoma, Ewing's sarcoma, osteosarcoma, aneurysmal bone cyst, infantile myofibromatosis, Gaucher's disease, and chronic recurrent multifocal osteomyelitis.

Sacrococcygeal teratoma
Sacrococcygeal teratoma is the most frequent congenital tumor and typically affects neonates. These tumors may be isolated or associated with anorectal malformations and caudal agenesis in the setting of the Currarino triad [38]. The lesion is solid or partly cystic and is usually huge, sometimes as large as or even larger than the newborn itself. Although the majority of teratomas in infancy and childhood

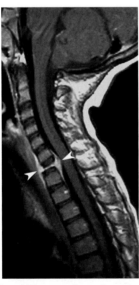

Fig. 16. Eosinophilic granuloma in a 5-year-old boy. Gadolinium-enhanced, sagittal T1-weighted MR image shows collapse of the C7 vertebral body associated with markedly enhancing pathologic tissue that completely replaces bone marrow and extends anteriorly in the prevertebral space and posteriorly into the epidural space (*arrowheads*). The adjacent disks are completely spared.

are benign, there is a tendency for malignant transformation as the child gets older [39]. Mature forms are characterized by the association of parenchymal tissue, fat, and calcifications. Immature teratomas lack fatty tissue and may show elevated growth rate and metastases. Sacrococcygeal teratomas are categorized into four groups: (I) external mass without a significant presacral component, (II) prevailingly external lesion with a relatively significant intrapelvic component, (III) prevailingly intrapelvic mass, and (IV) intrapelvic mass without external portions.

Malignant bone tumors

Ewing's sarcoma
Ewing's sarcoma is the most common primary bone tumor in children. Fewer than 10% are primitively located in the spine [40], where they account for 50% of pediatric spinal malignancies [1]. The lumbosacral region is the most common location [39,40], accounting for two thirds of cases in our series [1]. Presentation is by the end of the first decade of life [1] with local pain, radiculopathy, and signs of spinal cord compression, commonly associated with nonspecific systemic signs including fever, weight loss, anemia, and increased erythrosedimentation rate. Histologically, there is hypercellularity composed of small rounded cells with prominent nucleus and scant cytoplasm, similar to neuroblastomas and PNETs. Most tumors cause vertebral osteolysis associated with a soft tissue mass that may involve the paravertebral spaces and the intraspinal epidural compartment. Ewing's sarcoma may spread across the disk space to the adjacent vertebra, mimicking infection [39].

Conventional radiographs and CT show a permeative osteolytic mass containing sclerotic and calcific depositions. Vertebral collapse may occur (Fig. 17). Periosteal reactions are uncommon. CT and MR imaging show the extraosseous soft tumor components, which are typically abundant (see Fig. 17) and tend to envelope the affected bone, producing a sort of tumoral coating to the involved vertebrae that represents a useful diagnostic finding. Extradural extension and thecal sac compression are exquisitely depicted by MR imaging. The mass is iso- to hypointense on T1- and T2-weighted images, and contrast enhancement can vary from marked to absent (see Fig. 17).

Osteosarcoma
Only 4% of osteosarcomas primarily involve the spine in the general population, and the tumor is rare in the pediatric age group [41]. In the sacrum, the tumor prevailingly originates from the body and sacral ala, whereas nonsacral osteosarcomas typically (79%) arise in the posterior elements

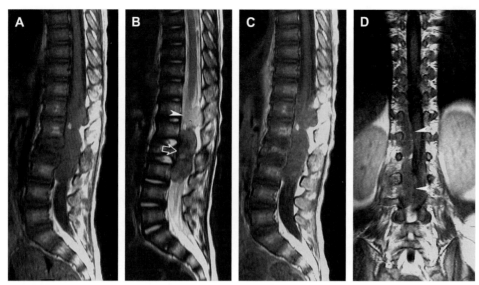

Fig. 17. Ewing's sarcoma in a 3-year-old boy. (*A*) Sagittal T1-weighted MR image shows L2 vertebral body collapse and a huge isointense intraspinal mass extending from T12 to L3. (*B*) Sagittal T2-weighted MR image shows the intraspinal mass with two components: one that is hyperintense at T12-L1 (*arrowhead*) and a larger one that is hypointense at L1-L3 (*open arrow*). (*C*) Gadolinium-enhanced, sagittal T1-weighted MR image shows lack of enhancement of the intraspinal portion. The collapsed L2 vertebral body remains isointense with the adjacent vertebrae. (*D*) Gadolinium-enhanced, coronal T1-weighted MR image confirms the extradural location of the soft tissue mass (*arrowheads*).

with partial body involvement [41]. Sclerotic and lytic lesions are found, often in association with soft tissue masses, mimicking Ewing's sarcomas and osteoblastomas.

Lymphoma and leukemia

Vertebral involvement from leukemia and lymphoma is common and can be primary or secondary. MR imaging findings include diffuse involvement of the vertebra with replacement of normal bone marrow signal intensity with an abnormal intermediate signal intensity resulting from neoplastic infiltration. Lymphomas also cause epidural mass formation, sometimes mimicking disk herniation, and cortical destruction with vertebral collapse. On MR imaging, hemolymphoproliferative tissue is low signal on T1- and T2-weighted images [42].

Tumors of the epidural spaces

Extraosseous sarcomas

Extraosseous sarcomas are a subset of small round cell tumors, histologically and ultrastructurally similar to the skeletal form of Ewing's sarcoma and PNETs, which originate from the meninges and grow within the extradural space without evidence of bone involvement, with possible extension to the paravertebral spaces through the neural foramina [43–45]. Affected patients present with signs of spinal cord compression that may be progressive.

On neuroimaging, these hypercellular tumors are iso- to hyperdense on unenhanced CT, slightly hypointense on T1-weighted images, and iso- to hypointense in T2-weighted images. Contrast enhancement is marked and may be heterogeneous due to necrotic-cystic changes. Differentiation from a classical Ewing's sarcoma is based on the absence of detectable vertebral involvement (Fig. 18).

Lymphoma and leukemia

Chloromas are the most common extraosseous spinal masses in patients with acute myeloid leukemia. These highly vascularized lesions are composed of immature granulocytes and are therefore also called granulocytic sarcomas. On MR imaging, they are iso- to hyperintense on T1-weighted images, iso- to hypointense on T2-weighted images, and show moderate to marked gadolinium enhancement. Extreme responsiveness to chemotherapy contraindicates surgery, with the exception of masses causing acute spinal cord compression [1].

Lymphomas may involve the epidural space selectively, often in the setting of multisystem disease. These epidural, strongly enhancing masses displace the epidural fat and may cause thecal sac and spinal cord compression (Fig. 19).

Germ cell tumors

Germ cell lineage tumors include germinomas, nongerminomatous tumors (embryonal carcinomas,

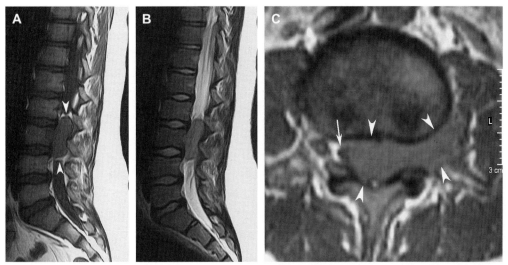

Fig. 18. Extraosseous sarcoma in an 11-year-old boy. (A) Sagittal T1-weighted MR image shows intraspinal mass centered at L3 and surrounded by epidural fat (*arrowheads*). (B) On sagittal T2-weighted MR image, the lesion is hypointense to CSF. The vertebral bodies are uninvolved. (C) Gadolinium-enhanced, axial T1-weighted MR image shows extradural mass extending into the enlarged left intervertebral foramen (*arrowheads*). The thecal sac is markedly compressed and displaced to the right (*arrow*).

yolk sac tumors, choriocarcinomas, and teratomas), and mixed tumors. Although rarely reported in the literature [46], the epidural space at the lumbosacral level is not an unlikely location of nongerminomatous germ cell tumors (30% of epidural space tumors in our series) [1].

Isolated germ cell tumors give nonspecific MR imaging findings (Fig. 20), but association of a large solid mass with sacrococcygeal agenesis is strongly suggestive. Germ cell tumor markers, such as β–human-chorionic gonadotropin, α-fetoprotein, and placental alkaline-phosphatase, are helpful adjuncts in the diagnostic workup.

Cellular schwannoma
Cellular schwannoma is a variety of peripheral nerve sheath tumor showing a predominantly compact cellular growth. The extent of the soft tissue

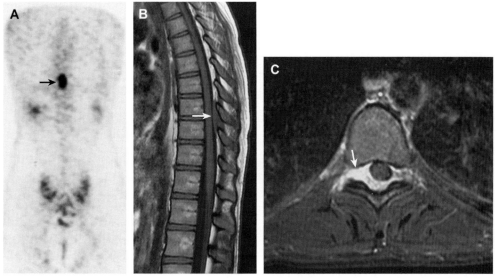

Fig. 19. B-cell lymphoma in 17-year-old renal transplant recipient. (A) Radionuclide bone scan shows markedly increased uptake at T9 (*arrow*). (B) Sagittal T1-weighted MR image shows posterior epidural soft tissue mass at T9-10 (*arrow*). (C) Gadolinium-enhanced, fat-suppressed axial T1-weighted MR image shows enhancing tissue extending into right neural foramen (*arrow*).

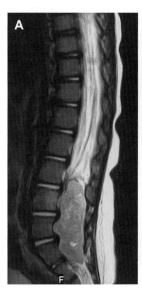
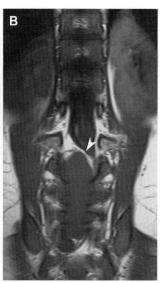

Fig. 20. Yolk sac tumor in a 17-month-old girl. (*A*) Sagittal T2-weighted MR image shows a heterogeneous lesion causing scalloping of the L4-S1 vertebral bones. (*B*) Coronal T1-weighted MR image shows a huge soft tissue mass filling the spinal canal at lumbosacral level. Extradural location is revealed by the typical meniscus appearance of the displaced epidural fat (*arrowhead*).

mass, frequent evidence of bony erosion and destruction, and confusing histologic features may produce the erroneous impression of a malignant tumor [47,48]. There is no association with neurofibromatosis. The nerve roots of the posterior neck, mediastinum, and retroperitoneum are the most common sites of origin. Most reported patients have been adults [49]. In the spine, we have seen a case of a large epidural soft tissue mass obliterating the lumbar spinal canal [1]. The MR imaging appearance was that of a huge soft tissue mass giving homogeneous isointense signal with cord on T1- and T2-weighted images and enhancing moderately and homogeneously. The lesion extended into the neural foramina, which might have supported a diagnosis of nerve sheath tumor. The diagnosis was histologic.

Extraspinal tumors with spinal invasion

Neuroblastoma
Neuroblastomas originate from the neural crests at the adrenal glands (40% of cases), the paravertebral

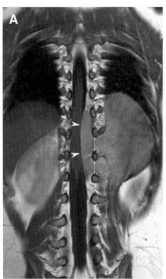
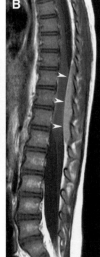
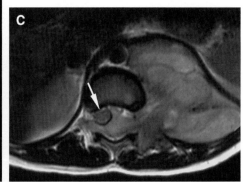

Fig. 21. Neuroblastoma in a 2-year-old girl. (*A*) Gadolinium-enhanced, coronal T1-weighted MR image shows large thoracoabdominal mass penetrating into the spinal canal through two enlarged neural foramina (*double arrows*) causing spinal cord compression (*arrowheads*). (*B*) Gadolinium-enhanced, sagittal T1-weighted MR image confirms an epidural tumor mass causing spinal cord compression (*arrowheads*). (*C*) Axial T2-weighted MR image shows a laterally displaced spinal cord (*arrow*) without signal abnormalities.

sympathetic chains (25% of cases), the organ of Zuckerkandl, and the carotid and aortic glomi. They are the most common non-CNS solid tumors in the pediatric age group and typically affect children younger than 5 years of age [1]. The tumor mass is typically huge and may show extensive necrotic-hemorrhagic areas and calcification. Histologically, there is a regular pattern of small rounded cells with high nuclear-to-cytoplasmic ratio, similar to Ewing's sarcomas and PNETs. There is a continuous histologic spectrum ranging from high-grade forms (neuroblastoma) through intermediate forms (ganglioneuroblastomas) to low-grade forms (ganglioneuroma). Tumor maturation from high to low grade may occur spontaneously or as a consequence of medical treatment. There are no radiologic criteria permitting a differentiation of high-grade from low-grade tumors. The clinical presentation is variable depending on the variable location and size of the mass; however, neurologic signs typically ensue with intraspinal extension and thecal sac compression. A rare, but specific, presentation of neuroblastomas is Kinsbourne syndrome, affecting 1% to 2% of all infants with neuroblastoma and characterized by opsoclonus, myoclonus, ataxia, and irritability [50].

Neuroblastomas originating from the paravertebral sympathetic chains typically display a "dumb-bell" growth through one or more neural foramina, extending a variably sized component into the spinal canal (Fig. 21) [51]. These intraspinal extradural masses may compress and displace the thecal sac and spinal cord, often extending along variable metameres cranial and caudad to the entrance foramen, as seen on the coronal planes. The mass is usually hypointense on T1-weighted images and iso- to hypointense on T2-weighted images due to high cellularity and nuclear-to-cytoplasmatic ratio. Necrotic-cystic change, hemorrhage, and calcification result in heterogeneous signal behavior. Contrast enhancement is usually marked. MR imaging detects compression and dislocation of the spinal cord, with possible intramedullary T2 hyperintensities reflecting compression-related myelopathy.

Nerve sheath tumors

Schwannomas and neurofibromas are known for their typical dumb-bell development through an enlarged neural foramen. They may occur in isolation or in association with neurofibromatosis.

Extramedullary erythropoiesis

Thalassemic patients may have multiple paravertebral masses or epidural masses resulting from extramedullary hematopoiesis. These masses are a result of compensatory hypertrophy of hematopoietic bone marrow at level of the costovertebral

junctions or vertebral bodies. Typically, there are paravertebral masses that abut the external orifice of the neural foramina without extending into the spinal canal [52]; however, spinal cord compression from epidural masses has been reported [52,53].

References

[1] Tortori-Donati P, Rossi A, Biancheri R, et al. Tumors of the spine and spinal cord. In: Tortori-Donati P, editor. Pediatric neuroradiology. Berlin: Springer Verlag; 2005. p. 1609–51.

[2] Koeller KK, Rosenblum RS, Morrison AL. Neoplasms of the spinal cord and filum terminale: radiologic-pathologic correlation. Radiographics 2000;20:1721–49.

[3] Aysun S, Cinbis M, Ozcan OE. Intramedullary astrocytoma presenting as spinal muscular atrophy. J Child Neurol 1993;8:354–6.

[4] Felice KJ, DiMario FJ. Cervicomedullary astrocytoma simulating a neuromuscular disorder. Pediatr Neurol 1999;20:78–80.

[5] Prasad VS, Basha A, Prasad BC, et al. Intraspinal tumour presenting as hydrocephalus in childhood. Childs Nerv Syst 1994;10:156–7.

[6] Kahan H, Sklar EM, Post MJ, et al. MR characteristics of histopathologic subtypes of spinal ependymoma. AJNR Am J Neuroradiol 1996;17:143–50.

[7] Merchant TE, Nguyen D, Thompson SJ, et al. High-grade pediatric spinal cord tumors. Pediatr Neurosurg 1999;30:1–5.

[8] Hamburger C, Buttner A, Weis S. Ganglioglioma of the spinal cord: report of two rare cases and review of the literature. Neurosurgery 1997;41:1410–6.

[9] Houten JK, Weiner HL. Pediatric intramedullary spinal cord tumors: special considerations. J Neurooncol 2000;47:225–30.

[10] Patel U, Pinto RS, Miller DC, et al. MR of spinal cord ganglioglioma. AJNR Am J Neuroradiol 1998;19:879–87.

[11] Castillo M. Gangliogliomas: ubiquitous or not? AJNR Am J Neuroradiol 1998;19:807–9.

[12] Nemoto Y, Inoue Y, Tashiro T, et al. Intramedullary spinal cord tumors: significance of associated hemorrhage at MR imaging. Radiology 1992;182:793–6.

[13] Wippold FJ II, Smirniotopoulos JG, Moran CJ, et al. MR imaging of myxopapillary ependymoma: findings and value to determine extent of tumor and its relations to intraspinal structures. AJR Am J Roentgenol 1995;165:1263–7.

[14] Cihangiroglu M, Hartker FW, Lee M, et al. Intraosseous sacral myxopapillary ependymoma and the differential diagnosis of sacral tumors. J Neuroimaging 2001;11:330–2.

[15] Alameda F, Lloreta J, Ferrer MD, et al. Clear-cell meningioma of the lumbosacral spine with choroid features. Ultrastruct Pathol 1999;23:51–8.

[16] Lee W, Chang KH, Choe G, et al. MR imaging features of clear-cell meningioma with diffuse leptomeningeal seeding. AJNR Am J Neuroradiol 2000;21:130–2.

[17] Yu KB, Lim MK, Kim HJ, et al. Clear-cell meningioma: CT and MR imaging findings in two cases involving the spinal canal and cerebellopontine angle. Korean J Radiol 2002;3:125–9.

[18] Zorludemir S, Scheithauer BW, Hirose T, et al. Clear cell meningioma: a clinicopathologic study of a potentially aggressive variant of meningioma. Am J Surg Pathol 1995;19:493–505.

[19] Tamiya T, Nakashima H, Ono Y, et al. Spinal atypical teratoid/rhabdoid tumor in an infant. Pediatr Neurosurg 2000;32:145–9.

[20] Tortori-Donati P, Fondelli MP, Rossi A, et al. Atypical teratoid rhabdoid tumors of the central nervous system in infancy: neuroradiologic findings. International Journal of Neuroradiology 1997;3:327–38.

[21] Kleihues P, Cavenee WK. Pathology and genetics, tumors of the nervous system. Lyon (France): IARC Press; 1997. p. 207–14.

[22] Albrecht CF, Weiss E, Schulz-Schaeffer WJ, et al. Primary intraspinal primitive neuroectodermal tumor: report of two cases and review of the literature. J Neurooncol 2003;61:113–20.

[23] Deme S, Ang LC, Skaf G, et al. Primary intramedullary primitive neuroectodermal tumor of the spinal cord: case report and review of the literature. Neurosurgery 1997;41:1417–20.

[24] Yavuz AA, Yaris N, Yavuz MN, et al. Primary intraspinal primitive neuroectodermal tumor: case report of a tumor arising from the sacral spinal nerve root and review of the literature. Am J Clin Oncol 2002;25:135–9.

[25] Tortori-Donati P, Rossi A, Cama A. Spinal dysraphism: a review of neuroradiological features with embryological correlations and proposal for a new classification. Neuroradiology 2000;42:471–91.

[26] Hayes CW, Conway WF, Sundaram M. Misleading aggressive MR imaging appearance of some benign musculoskeletal lesions. Radiographics 1992;12:1119–34.

[27] Woods ER, Martel W, Mandell SH, et al. Reactive soft-tissue mass associated with osteoid osteoma: correlation of MR imaging features with pathologic findings. Radiology 1993;186:221–5.

[28] Davies M, Cassar-Pullicino VN, Davies AM, et al. The diagnostic accuracy of MR imaging in osteoid osteoma. Skeletal Radiol 2002;31:559–69.

[29] Liu PT, Chivers FS, Roberts CC, et al. Imaging of osteoid osteoma with dynamic gadolinium-enhanced MR imaging. Radiology 2003;227:691–700.

[30] Jackson RP, Reckling FW, Mantz FA. Osteoid osteoma and osteoblastoma. Clin Orthop 1977;128:303–13.

[31] Beltran J, Simon DC, Levy M, et al. Aneurysmal bone cysts: MR imaging at 1.5 T. Radiology 1986;158:689–90.

[32] Munk PL, Helms CA, Holt RG, et al. MR imaging of aneurysmal bone cysts. AJR Am J Roentgenol 1989;153:99–101.

[33] Tsai JC, Dalinka MK, Fallon MD, et al. Fluid-fluid level: a nonspecific finding in tumors of bone and soft tissue. Radiology 1990;175:779–82.

[34] Papagelopoulos PJ, Currier BL, Shaughnessy WJ, et al. Aneurysmal bone cyst of the spine: management and outcome. Spine 1998;23:621–8.

[35] Ladisch S, Jaffe ES. The histiocytoses. In: Pizzo PA, Poplack DG, editors. Principles and practice of pediatric oncology. Philadelphia: Lippincott; 1989. p. 491–504.

[36] Ippolito E, Farsetti P, Tudisco C. Vertebra plana: long term follow-up in 5 patients. J Bone Joint Surg Am 1984;66-A:1364–8.

[37] Garg S, Mehta S, Dormans JP. An atypical presentation of Langerhans cell histiocytosis of the cervical spine in a child. Spine 2003;28:E445–8.

[38] Currarino G, Coln D, Votteler T. Triad of anorectal, sacral, and presacral anomalies. AJR Am J Roentgenol 1981;137:395–8.

[39] Diel J, Ortiz O, Losada RA, et al. The sacrum: pathologic spectrum, multimodality imaging, and subspecialty approach. Radiographics 2001;21:83–104.

[40] Venkateswaran L, Rodriguez-Galindo C, Merchant TE, et al. Primary Ewing tumor of the vertebrae: clinical characteristics, prognostic factors, and outcome. Med Pediatr Oncol 2001;37:30–5.

[41] Ilaslan H, Sundaram M, Unni KK, et al. Primary vertebral osteosarcoma: imaging findings. Radiology 2004;230:697–702.

[42] Ginsberg LE, Leeds NE. Neuroradiology of leukemia. AJR Am J Roentgenol 1995;165:525–34.

[43] Allam K, Sze G. MR of primary extraosseous Ewing sarcoma. AJNR Am J Neuroradiol 1994;15:305–7.

[44] Scazzeri F, Prosetti D, Ferrito G, et al. Un caso di sarcoma di Ewing extraosseo. Rivista di Neuroradiologia 1996;9:623–5 [in Italian].

[45] Shin JH, Lee HK, Rhim SC, et al. Spinal epidural extraskeletal Ewing sarcoma: MR findings in two cases. AJNR Am J Neuroradiol 2001;22:795–8.

[46] Choi SJ, Choi HJ, Hong JT, et al. Intraspinal extradural teratoma mimicking neural sheath tumor in infant. Childs Nerv Syst 2004;20:123–6.

[47] Woodruff JM, Godwin TA, Erlandson RA, et al. Cellular schwannoma: a variety of schwannoma sometimes mistaken for a malignant tumor. Am J Surg Pathol 1981;5:733–44.

[48] Fletcher CD, Davies SE, McKee PH. Cellular schwannoma: a distinct pseudosarcomatous entity. Histopathology 1987;11:21–35.

[49] White W, Shiu MH, Rosenblum MK, et al. Cellular schwannoma: a clinicopathologic study of 57 patients and 58 tumors. Cancer 1990;66:1266–75.

[50] Veneselli E, Conte M, Biancheri R, et al. Effect of steroid and high-dose immunoglobulin therapy on opsoclonus-myoclonus syndrome occurring in neuroblastoma. Med Pediatr Oncol 1998;30: 15–7.

[51] Slovis TL, Meza MP, Cushing B, et al. Thoracic neuroblastoma: what is the best imaging modality for evaluating extent of disease? Pediatr Radiol 1997;27:273–5.

[52] Chourmouzi D, Pistevou-Gompaki K, Plataniotis G, et al. MRI findings of extramedullary haemopoiesis. Eur Radiol 2001;11: 1803–6.

[53] Dibbern DA Jr, Loevner LA, Lieberman AP, et al. MR of thoracic cord compression caused by epidural extramedullary hematopoiesis in myelodysplastic syndrome. AJNR Am J Neuroradiol 1997;18:363–6.

NEUROIMAGING
CLINICS
OF NORTH AMERICA

Neuroimag Clin N Am 17 (2007) 37–55

ELSEVIER
SAUNDERS

Demyelinating and Infectious Diseases of the Spinal Cord

Majda M. Thurnher, MD*, Fabiola Cartes-Zumelzu, MD,
Christina Mueller-Mang, MD

- Demyelinating diseases of the spinal cord
  Multiple sclerosis
  Devic's neuromyelitis optica
  Transverse myelitis
  Acute disseminated encephalomyelitis
  Subacute combined degeneration
  AIDS-associated myelopathy
- Spinal cord infections
  Bacterial myelitis and spinal cord abscess
  Tuberculosis
  Toxoplasmosis
- Summary
- References

Spinal cord diseases generally have distinctive clinical findings that reflect dysfunction of particular sensory or motor tracts. The abnormalities on MR images reflect the pathologic changes that occur in the affected pathways. The complexity and the wide spectrum of diseases affecting the spinal cord require a profound knowledge of neuropathology and exactly tuned imaging strategies. This article describes and illustrates the clinical and imaging characteristics in various demyelinating and infectious conditions of the spinal cord.

Demyelinating diseases of the spinal cord

Multiple sclerosis

Multiple sclerosis (MS) is a chronic inflammatory demyelinating disease of the central nervous system (CNS). Recent data suggest that MS is a T-cell–mediated disease with secondary macrophage activation. The pathologic hallmark of MS is inflammatory demyelination, which can lead to irreversible tissue loss or partial demyelination in cases where reparative processes occur with subsequent remyelination. Three mechanisms of tissue injury in MS have been proposed: immunologic, excitotoxic, and metabolic [1]. The spinal cord is frequently involved in MS, with cord lesions found in up to 99% of autopsy cases [2,3]. The first pathologic descriptions of the macroscopic distribution of MS lesions in the spinal cord were by Carswell in 1838 [4] and Cruveilhier in 1841 [5]. In 70% to 80% of patients who have MS, cord abnormalities are detected on T2-weighted MR images [6]. MS spinal cord abnormalities can be divided into three main types: (1) focal, well demarcated areas of high signal intensity on T2-WI; (2) diffuse abnormalities seen as poorly demarcated areas of increased signal intensity on T2-WI; and (3) spinal cord atrophy and axonal loss.

Focal lesions

Macroscopically, spinal cord lesions appear elongated in the direction of the long axis of the cord and vary in length from a few millimeters to lesions that extend over multiple segments [7]. MR imaging is the most sensitive technique for detecting MS

Department of Radiology, Neuroradiology Section, Medical University of Vienna, Waehringer Guertel 18-20, Vienna A-1090, Austria
* Corresponding author.
E-mail address: majda.thurnher@meduniwien.ac.at (M.M. Thurnher).

doi:10.1016/j.nic.2006.12.002

lesions in the brain and spinal cord. Its role as a tool in the diagnosis and longitudinal monitoring of patients who have MS has been well established in numerous studies [8–12]. The recent introduction of the McDonald [11] criteria has further strengthened the role of MR imaging in the diagnosis of MS. MS plaques are best seen with T2-weighted MR sequences and are hyperintense on T2-WI and iso-hypointense on T1-weighted MR images. Spinal cord demyelinating plaques present as well circumscribed foci of increased T2 signal that asymmetrically involve the spinal cord parenchyma. They are characteristically peripherally located, are less than two vertebral segments in length, and occupy less than half the cross-sectional area of the cord. On sagittal sections, plaques have a cigar shape and may be located centrally, anteriorly, and dorsally. On axial MR images, the lesions located in the lateral segments have a wedge shape with the basis at the cord surface or a round shape if there is no contact with the cord surface (Fig. 1). The distribution of MS lesions in the spinal cord closely corresponds to venous drainage areas. Cord swelling is usually found only in the relapsing-remitting form of MS [12–14]. Because acute lesions are associated with transient breakdown of the blood–brain barrier, enhancement may be seen on postcontrast images (Figs. 2 and 3). The incidence of enhancing lesions is significantly lower than in the brain [7]. Sixty-two percent of the plaques occur in the cervical spinal cord. Chronic foci of hypointensity on T1-WI images, known in the brain as "black holes," are not present in the spinal cord [15].

Diffuse abnormalities

Diffuse abnormalities are more common in primary progressive MS and secondary progressive MS. Diffuse signal changes of the spinal cord are recognized on images as mild intramedullary hyperintensities on T2-weighted MR images (Fig. 4).

Spinal cord atrophy

In addition to plaques and diffuse spinal cord abnormalities, spinal cord atrophy has been recognized for many years (Fig. 5). Axonal degeneration, or an alternative atrophic process, may be responsible for spinal cord atrophy in MS. One recent study has shown that the degree of atrophy varies

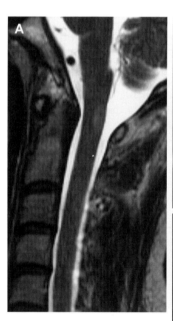
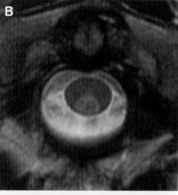
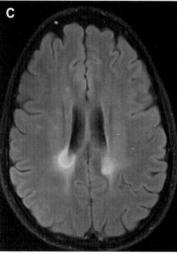

Fig. 1. Typical MS lesion in the cervical spinal cord. (*A*) Sagittal T2-weighted MR image showing hyperintense, dorsally located spinal cord lesion at the C2 level. (*B*) On axial T2-weighted MR image, a hyperintense, wedge-shaped lesion is located in the dorsal aspect of the spinal cord lesion, occupying less than half the cross-sectional area of the cord. (*C*) Axial fluid-attenuated, inversion-recovery–weighted MR image of the brain in the same patient showing hyperintense periventricular white matter lesions consistent with MS lesions.

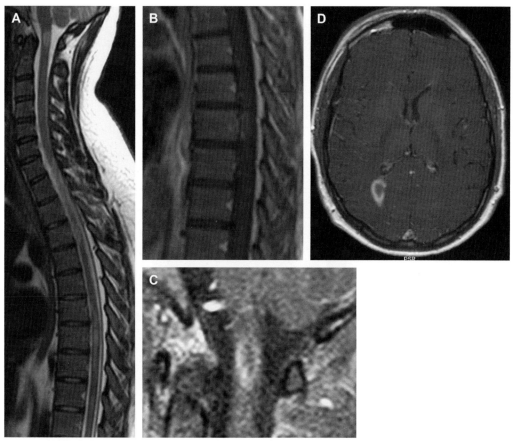

Fig. 2. Multiple spinal cord focal lesions in a patient who has MS. (*A*) Sagittal T2-weighted MR image showing several high-signal-intensity lesions in the spinal cord at levels C1/C2, T3, and from T6 to T8, consistent with spinal MS manifestation. (*B*) A sagittal gadolinium-enhanced, T1-weighted MR image demonstrating enhancement of the lesion at the T7 level, consistent with acute inflamed MS plaque. (*C*) Ring enhancement of the lesions located at the C2 level is observed on a sagittal postcontrast, T1-weighted MR image. (*D*) Axial T1-weighted, contrast-enhanced MR image of the brain showing a ring-like enhancing lesion in the left occipital white matter lesions.

in different parts of the cord, being more prominent in upper parts of the cord [16]. Studies have also shown that spinal cord atrophy correlates with clinical disability [16]. Analysis of the amount of atrophy revealed a correlation between upper cervical cord and cerebral white matter atrophy and an expanded disability status scale [17]. Significant cerebral and spinal cord volume reductions have been found in all patient subgroups of MS compared with control subjects [17]. Higher rates of atrophy have been reported in relapsing-remitting MS than in secondary progressive forms of the disease [17]. Plaques associated with cord atrophy are more likely to occur with the relapsing-progressive form of MS.

Axonal loss

Postmortem studies have shown convincingly that cord damage is not limited to lesions visible on T2-WI [18]. According to the neuropathologic studies about MS of the spinal cord, axonal loss can be found in 60% to 70% of chronic MS lesions. Magnetic Resonance Spectroscopy studies have shown reduced N-acetyl aspartate in areas of the cord that were normal on conventional MR images. Significant abnormalities in normal-appearing spinal cord have also been observed [19]. Decreased small fiber density was found in one study in the lateral column of the cervical spinal cord of patients who have MS compared with control subjects [20]. Data from recent neuropathologic studies suggest that extensive axonal damage occurs during plaque formation soon after the onset of demyelination [21]. Furthermore, during that process, significant axonal injury is found in the normal white matter. Ongoing, low-burning axonal destruction has also been found in inactive demyelinated lesions in the brain [21].

The entire spinal cord should be imaged in patients who have spinal symptoms and who have

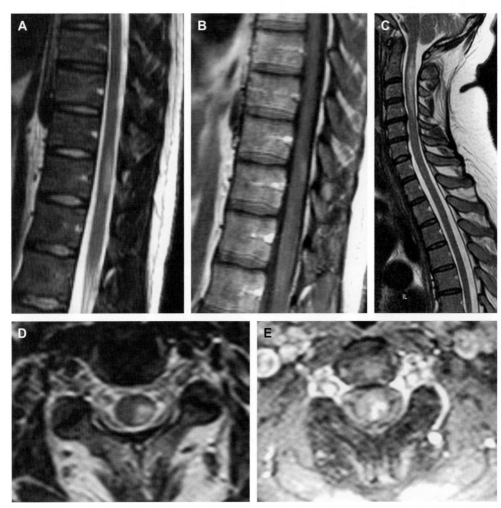

Fig. 3. Active (enhancing) focal spinal cord lesion in two patients who have MS. (*A*) Sagittal T2-weighted MR image of the thoracic spine showing a focal hyperintense spinal cord lesion consistent with a focal MS lesion in the spinal cord. (*B*) On sagittal postcontrast, T1-weighted MR image, subtle nodular enhancement of the MS lesion is observed. (*C, D*) In another patient, a wedge-shaped, high-signal-intensity lesion located in the lateral aspect of the cord (*D*) extending from C2 to C4 with mild cord expansion is demonstrated on a sagittal T2-weighted MR image (*C*). (*E*) Peripheral enhancement of the lesion is demonstrated on an axial postcontrast T1-weighted MR image with fat suppression.

a known or presumptive diagnosis of MS. Slice thickness should not exceed 3 mm, with a maximum interslice gap of 10% [10]. The imaging protocol should include the following sequences: sagittal T2-WI, T1-WI, axial T2-WI for exact anatomic location of the lesion, and contrast-enhanced T1-WI. Studies have shown the superiority of short-tau inversion-recovery sequences to Fast Spin Echo sequences in the detection of MS lesions in the spinal cord (Fig. 6) [22,23]. Fast fluid inversion recovery was rated unsatisfactory [22].

The value of spinal MR imaging in the differentiation of MS from other inflammatory or cerebrovascular disorders has been evaluated in a recent study [24]. Specificity, sensitivity, and positive and negative predictive values for MR imaging

were calculated for 66 patients who had other neurologic diseases and 25 patients who had MS. Brain images were abnormal in all patients who had MS but in only 65% of patients who had other brain disorders. Spinal cord abnormality was found in 92% of patients who had MS but in only 6% of patients who had other diseases. With the combination of brain and spinal cord MR imaging in that study, the accuracy of differentiating MS from other disorders reached 95% based on the criteria of Paty and colleagues [25], 93% based on the criteria of Fazekas and colleagues [26], and 93% based on the criteria of Barkhof and colleagues [27].

Diffusion-weighted MR imaging (DWI) has been increasingly used for the evaluation of spinal cord

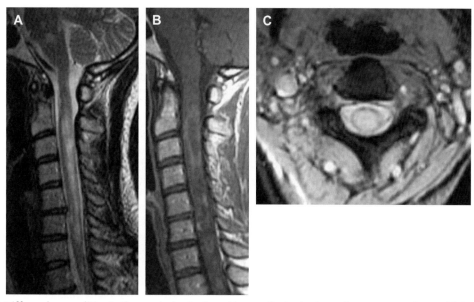

Fig. 4. Diffuse abnormalities in the cervical spinal cord in a patient who has primary progressive multiple sclerosis. (*A*) Sagittal T2-weighted MR-image showing increased signal intensity on T2-WI in the cervical spinal cord, extending to multiple segments with cord enlargement. (*B*) Sagittal T1-weighted, gadolinium-enhanced MR images showing diffuse, poorly demarcated enhancement of the spinal cord lesions. (*C*) On axial T2-weighted MR image, the lesion involves almost the whole area of the spinal cord.

diseases, especially in spinal cord ischemia [28,29]. Clark and colleagues [30] were the first to use a conventional, cardiac-gated, navigation diffusion-sensitized spin-echo sequence for in vivo DW imaging of the spinal cord. MS lesions were found to have increased rates of diffusivity, with a significantly higher isotropic diffusion coefficient, compared with healthy control subjects. Differences in diffusion anisotropy did not reach statistical significance. The decrease in anisotropy is probably due to several factors, such as loss of myelin from white matter fiber tracts, expansion of the extracellular space fraction, and perilesional inflammatory edema. Reduced anisotropy is also seen in MS brain lesions [31–33]. A large standard deviation in the lesion values was observed by Clark and colleagues, which could be explained by lesion heterogeneity. On postmortem high-resolution MR imaging of the spinal cord in MS, two main types of lesions have been found: lesions with marked signal intensity (SI) changes that corresponded with complete demyelination and lesions with mild SI abnormalities where only partial demyelination was found histologically [34].

To assess whether diffusion tensor-derived measures of cord tissue damage are related to clinical disability, mean diffusivity (MD) and fractional anisotropy (FA) histograms were acquired from the cervical cords obtained from a large cohort of patients who had MS [35]. In that study, diffusion-weighted, echo planar images of the spinal cord and brain DW images were acquired from 44 patients who had MS and from 17 healthy control subjects. The study showed that average cervical cord FA was significantly lower in patients who had MS compared with control subjects. Good correlation was found between the average FA and average MD and the degree of disability. In another recently published study, axial diffusion tensor MR imaging (DTI) was performed in 24 patients who had relapsing-remitting MS and 24 age- and sex-matched control subjects [36]. FA and MD were calculated in the anterior, lateral, and posterior spinal cord bilaterally and in the central spinal cord at the C2-C3 level. Significantly lower FA values were found in the lateral, dorsal, and central parts of the normal-appearing white matter in patients who had MS. The results of this study show that significant changes in DTI metrics are present in the cervical spinal cord of patients who have MS in the absence of spinal cord signal abnormality at conventional MR examination [36]. The exact value of DW imagining and DTI in MS of the spinal cord has not been completely evaluated [37].

Studies have been performed to evaluate the usefulness of T1 relaxation time and magnetization transfer ratio [38–40]. In one study of 90 patients who had MS and 20 control subjects, reduced histogram magnetization transfer ratio values were found in patients who had MS [39]. Although the results were encouraging, the long acquisition times are clinically questionable.

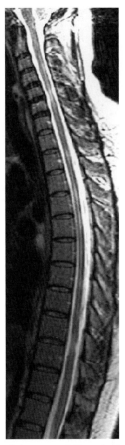

Fig. 5. A marked decrease of the spinal cord diameter is demonstrated on a sagittal T2-WI MR image in a patient who has MS.

Devic's neuromyelitis optica

Devic's neuromyelitis optica (DNMO) is a demyelinating disease characterized by bilateral visual disturbance and transverse myelopathy. It was first described in 1894 by Eugene Devic [41] in a woman who suffered from a bilateral optic neuritis and acute transverse myelitis. Pathologically, lesions are restricted to the optic nerves and spinal cord, with areas of necrosis of gray and white matter, cavitations, lack of inflammatory infiltrate, vascular hyalinization, and fibrosis [42]. Clinically, the disease may have a mono- or multiphasic course [43]. The nosology is not clear, and the reports from the literature are confusing. Historically, the disease was defined as a monophasic disorder consisting of fulminant bilateral optic neuritis and myelitis, occurring in close temporal association. Cases of DNMO that followed in the literature described more extensive findings, with a relapsing course, which raised the question of whether DNMO represents a separate syndrome or a variant of MS. One of the largest series published by a group from the Mayo Clinic included 71 patients who had DNMO [44]. Based on their findings, the initial definition was revised. Clinical characteristics, course, and prognosis have been evaluated further on 46 patients from 15 Italian MS centers [45]. Compared with patients who had MS, patients who had DNMO had a poor prognosis, higher age at onset, and a more sever clinical course. DNMO was most like to affect female patients. Corticosteroids are not helpful in DNMO, and the prognosis is poor. Cerebral spinal fluid (CSF) abnormalities include pleocytosis, high protein, and high albumin

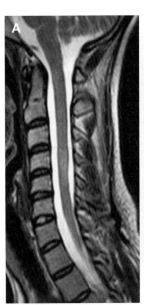
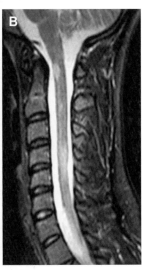

Fig. 6. Comparison of a T2-WI MR image and short-tau inversion-recovery MR image in the detection of spinal cord MS lesions. (*A*) On the sagittal T2-WI MR image of the cervical spinal cord, intramedullary high-signal-intensity lesions have been detected at the C2 and C4-C5 levels. Note the mild increase in signal intensity. (*B*) On the sagittal short-tau inversion-recovery MR sequence, focal lesions in the cord show a marked increase in signal intensity and are much more easily appreciated.

ratio levels [45]. The most common abnormality observed on MR images of the spinal cord is longitudinal, confluent lesions extending across five or more vertebral segments, with a hyperintensity on T2-weighted images (Fig. 7) [46,47]. Cord swelling and enhancement were present in 24 of 100 MR scans evaluated in one study [45]. In one study with nine patients diagnosed with possible DNMO in French hospitals, the authors observed that cord atrophy was associated with complete para- or quadriplegia, whereas cord swelling was associated with possible neurologic improvement [46]. Short inversion time inversion recovery techniques depict the lesions of the optic nerves in cases of presumed neuromyelitis optica [48]. MR imaging findings can be used to differentiate between DNMO and MS: In DNMO, no cerebral white matter lesions are present; spinal cord lesions are confluent and extend to multiple segments in DNMO, which is uncommon in MS; spinal cord atrophy is present in MS but is often described as part of the course of DNMO; and cranial nerves or cerebellar involvement are common in MS but are not present in DNMO [43–46]. The discovery of a novel serum autoantibody, NMO-IgG, with high sensitivity and specificity for DNMO, has significantly improved the early diagnosis of this severe demyelinating syndrome [49]. Clinical findings

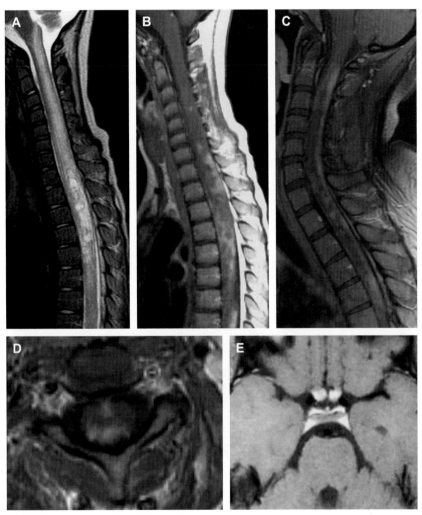

Fig. 7. Two patients who have DNMO. (*A*) Sagittal T2-weighted MR image of the cervico-thoracic spine showing longitudinal, confluent lesions extending across several vertebral segments with cord swelling. Note the cystic-appearing lesions at the T3–T6 level. (*B*) Patchy, confluent enhancement is observed on a postcontrast T1-WI MR image. (*C, D*) Sagittal (*C*) and axial (*D*) T1–weighted, gadolinium-enhanced MR images in another patient showing patchy enhancement of spinal cord abnormalities extending to multiple segments of the cervical cord. (*E*) On an axial-enhanced, T1-weighted MR image of the brain, marked enhancement of the optic nerves is demonstrated, consistent with bilateral optic neuritis in DNMO. (*Courtesy of* M. Castillo, MD, Chapel Hill, NC.)

that favor DNMO are higher age at onset and severe course [45]. Results from the recently published study challenge the classic belief of a sparing of the brain tissue in DNMO; compared with healthy control subjects, patients who had DNMO showed a reduced magnetization transfer ratio and increased mean diffusivity of the normal-appearing gray matter of the brain [50].

Transverse myelitis

The first cases of acute transverse myelitis (ATM) were described in 1882 by Bastian [51]. In 1922 and 1923, 200 cases of so-called "post-vaccination encephalomyelitis" were reported in Holland and England. It was in 1948 that the term ATM was used in reporting a case of severe myelopathy after pneumonia [52].

Transverse myelitis is a clinical syndrome characterized by bilateral motor, sensory, and autonomic disturbances [53]. About 50% of patients have paraparesis; 80% to 94% have numbness, paresthesias, and band-like dysesthesias; and all have bladder dysfunction [53]. The histopathologic features of TM include perivascular monocytic and lymphocytic infiltration, demyelination, and axonal injury [54]. TM may exist as part of a multifocal CNS disease; as a multi-systemic disease; or as an isolated, idiopathic entity. The immunopathogenesis of disease-associated TM is varied and includes vasculitis neurosarcoidosis, MS, and lupus. Several reports of

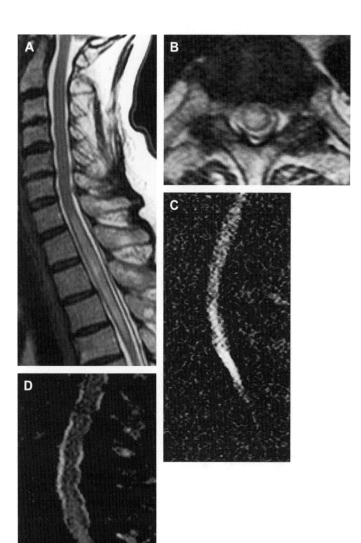

Fig. 8. ATM. (*A*) Sagittal T2-weighted MR image showing high-signal-intensity abnormality in the spinal cord lesion extending over several segments of the upper thoracic spine. (*B*) A focal, centrally located increased signal occupying more than two thirds of the cross-sectional area of the cord is demonstrated on the axial T2-weighted MR image. (*C*) On a sagittal, diffusion-weighted MR image performed using navigated interleaved multishot echo planar imaging (5-mm slice thickness, b max = 700 s/mm²), high signal indicates increased diffusion in the area of increased signal on T2-WI. (*D*) High signal was observed on the apparent diffusion coefficient map, suggesting a T2 shine-through effect rather than restricted diffusion in spinal cord areas affected by myelitis.

TM after vaccination have been published [55,56]. Recently, the term "parainfectious TM" has been introduced for TM cases with antecedent respiratory, gastrointestinal, or systemic illness [54]. A variety of immune stimuli (eg, molecular mimicry, superantigen-mediated immune activation) may trigger the immune system to injure the nervous system [54]. In a retrospective study of 288 patients who had TM, 45 (15.6%) met the criteria for idiopathic TM [57]. According to the published series, approximately one third of patients recover with little or no sequelae, one third are left with a moderate degree of permanent disability, and one third develop severe disability [58]. In 2002, the Transverse Myelitis Consortium Working Group proposed criteria for idiopathic ATM, with incorporation of CSF testing and MR imaging findings [58]. The criteria include (1) bilateral sensory, motor, or autonomic spinal cord dysfunction; (2) defined sensory level and bilateral signs and symptoms; (3) proof of inflammation within the spinal cord by MR imaging or CSF examination; (4) symptoms from onset to reach maximal deficit between few hours and 21 days; and (5) exclusion of extra-axial compressive etiology [58]. The thoracic spine is most commonly involved, and middle-aged adults are usually affected. MR imaging findings include focal, centrally located increased signal on T2-weighted MR images, usually occupying more than two thirds of the cross-sectional area of the cord (Fig. 8) [59]. This was observed in 88% of patients in a series of 17 patients who had idiopathic TM [60]. Usually, the signal abnormality extends more than three to four vertebral segments in length. Cord expansion may or may not be present; it was found in 47% in published series [59]. Enhancement is usually absent; when enhancement was present, two patterns have been described: moderate patchy enhancement or diffuse abnormal enhancement (Figs. 9 and 10) [57,60–62]. Enhancement was found in only 38% of cases of idiopathic TM in one series and in 47% and 53% in the two other series [57,59]. About 40% of TM cases display a normal MR imaging study [63]. MS is the most important differential diagnosis of TM. Signal abnormality located peripherally in the spinal cord that is less than two vertebral segments in length and occupying less than half the cross-sectional area of the cord favors a diagnosis of MS rather than TM [9].

There is growing evidence that the length of the lesion is likely important from a pathogenic and a prognostic standpoint. Patients who have acute partial transverse myelitis have signal abnormalities extending less than two segments on MR imaging, and patients who have complete longitudinally extensive transverse myelitis have abnormalities that extend to multiple segments (see Fig. 8). Patients

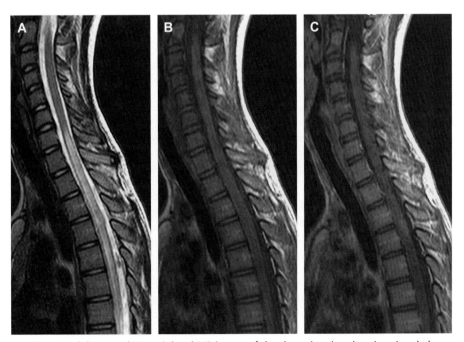

Fig. 9. Idiopathic ATM. (*A*) Sagittal T2-weighted MR image of the thoracic spine showing signal abnormality extending from T7 to the L2 vertebral segment. (*B*) The lesion is isointense to the spinal cord on sagittal T-weighted MR image. (*C*) Sagittal image showing focal enhancement in the cord.

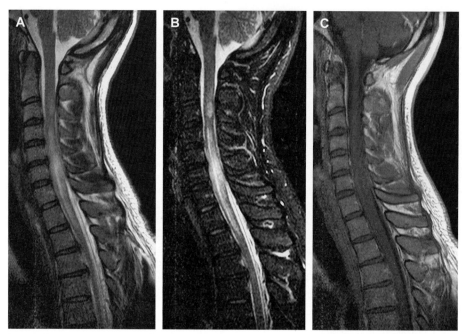

Fig. 10. A case of acute transverse myelitis in a patient who presented with sensory level. (*A, B*) T2-weighted (*A*) and sagittal short-tau inversion-recovery (*B*) MR images show high-signal-intensity abnormality in the cervical spinal cord extending from the C3 to the T1 level with cord swelling. (*C*) Sagittal gadolinium-enhanced, T1-weighted MR image showing moderate patchy enhancement.

in the first group are at higher risk for developing MS compared with those in the second group, where the risk is low [64].

DTI was recently used to characterize inflammatory processes of the spinal cord [65]. In cases of inflammatory myelitis, decreased FA values have been found in the region of a T2-weighted lesion and increased FA values in the lesion's boundaries. This pattern is different from that seen in invasive tumors, in which FA is low in peripheral regions of edema.

Novel biomarkers, such as cytokine interleukin-6 and collapsin response-mediator protein–5 are potentially useful prognostic indicators and markers of disease severity. The "idiopathic" form of ATM is rarely seen [66].

Acute disseminated encephalomyelitis

Acute disseminated encephalomyelitis (ADEM) is an acute demyelinating disorder of the CNS, usually occurring after infections and vaccinations. The most probable pathophysiology is an autoimmune response to myelin basic protein, triggered by infection or immunization. Although ADEM is usually considered a monophasic disease with a good prognosis, recurrent or multiphasic forms have been described [67–69]. ADEM seems to occur more frequently in children and young adults. The most frequent clinical symptoms include motor

deficits, sensory deficits, brain stem signs, and ataxia [9,64,65]. CSF findings are nonspecific, with oligoclonal bands detected in up to 65% of patients [67]. On MR imaging, ill-defined hyperintense lesions on T2-WI and hypointense lesions on T1-WI in the spinal cord can be recognized (Figs. 11 and 12) [70]. Lesions are usually large and extend over a long segment of the spinal cord with cord expansion (see Figs. 11 and 12). The thoracic cord is most commonly affected. Spinal cord involvement was reported in 71% of patients in one series [71]. All patients who had spinal involvement had cerebral lesions and signs of myelopathy [71]. The MR imaging appearance of ADEM is nonspecific and indistinguishable from other inflammatory lesions, particularly MS plaques. Many patients initially diagnosed with ADEM develop clinically definite MS upon long-term follow-up. In one clinical study, 35% of all adult patients initially diagnosed with ADEM developed MS over a mean observation period of 38 months [67]. Similar results have been reported in children, with 17 of 121 children initially diagnosed with ADEM later developing MS [71,72].

Some typical signs of ADEM have been described in the literature, such as involvement of the basal ganglia and thalamus, cortical lesions, and brainstem involvement. Combined clinical and radiologic studies failed to define reliable diagnostic

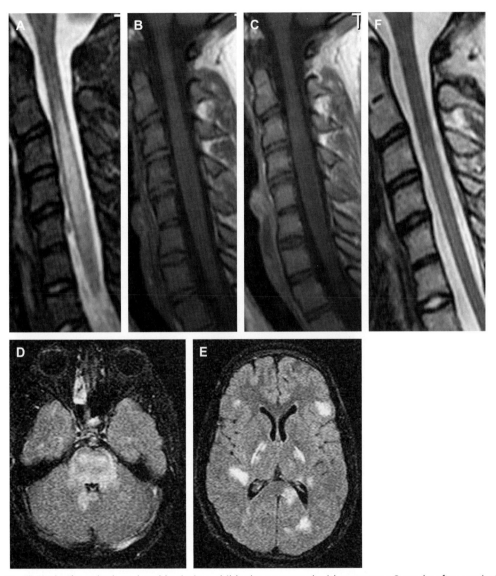

Fig. 11. ADEM in the spinal cord and brain in a child who presented with symptoms 2 weeks after respiratory illness. (*A*) On sagittal T2-WI MR image of the cervical spine, a high-signal-intensity lesion extending to multiple segments is observed in the cervical spinal cord. Note expansion of the cord. (*B, C*) No signal abnormality is noted on precontrast T1-WI MR image (*B*), and no enhancement is noted on postcontrast image (*C*). (*D, E*) Multiple high-signal-intensity lesions are present in the brain (pons, subcortical regions, basal ganglia) on axial T2-weighted MR images, consistent with ADEM. (*F*) Follow-up sagittal T2-weighted image a few weeks later shows complete resolution of MR imaging abnormalities.

criteria for the differentiation of a first episode of MS from monophasic ADEM [67,70]. As long as accurate diagnostic criteria have not been established, it is wise to use the term ADEM as a description of a clinical syndrome and not as a distinct entity, and the diagnosis of monophasic ADEM should be made with caution in all cases, especially in patients who have an onset in adulthood. Recently, magnetization transfer and diffusion tensor imaging have been used to characterize normal-appearing brain tissue and cervical spinal cord in patients who

have ADEM and to compare these images with images from control subjects and patients who had MS [73]. Normal-appearing brain tissue and cervical cord were spared except in the acute phase in patients who had ADEM, which was not true for patients who had MS.

Subacute combined degeneration

Vitamin B12 deficiency usually presents with pernicious anemia or various neuropsychiatric

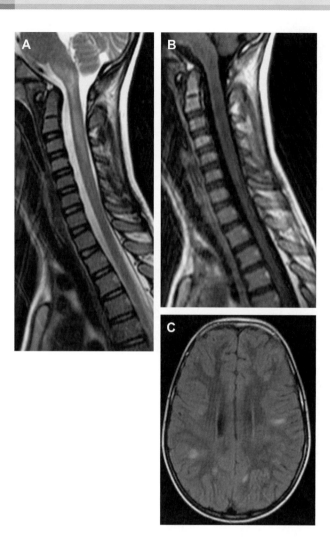

Fig. 12. ADEM in a 7-year-old child and involvement of the brain and cervical spinal cord. (*A*) Sagittal T2-weighted MR image showing a hyperintense cervical spinal cord lesion extending over multiple segments. (*B*) The lesion is hypointense on sagittal T1-weighted MR image. (*C*) Hyperintense lesions are present on axial fast fluid inversion recovery MR image in the subcortical regions, bilaterally in the parietal lobes, representing ADEM lesions.

manifestations. Patients with blind-loop syndrome, celiac disease, Crohn's disease, chronic pancreatic insufficiency, and vegetarians may develop B12 deficiency. Large-fiber neuropathy, myelopathy (subacute combined degeneration of the spinal cord), dementia, cerebellar ataxia, optic atrophy, psychosis, and mood disorders are the most common neuropsychiatric manifestations. The spinal cord involvement, called subacute combined degeneration, is clinically characterized by symmetric dysesthesia, disturbance of positional sense, spastic paraparesis, or tetraparesis [74]. Typical neuropathologic findings include a multifocal pattern of axonal loss and demyelination that is most prominent in the cervical and thoracic spinal cord [74]. Most commonly, the disease affects posterior columns, followed by the anterolateral and anterior tracts. In cases of subacute combined degeneration of the spinal cord, MR imaging demonstrates characteristic bilateral, hyperintense areas on T2-weighted images in the posterior columns of the cervical and

thoracic cord without contrast enhancement (Fig. 13) [75]. Signal abnormalities are common but may not be present in every patient. In one patient after gastrectomy, signal intensity abnormalities were observed in the posterior and anterior columns of the spinal cord [76]. A decrease in size was noted at the 9-month follow-up MR scan after appropriate therapy. Early diagnosis is essential to prevent significant cord damage. After vitamin B12 supplementation, patients show clinical and radiologic improvement. In one recently published case, contrast enhancement of the posterior columns and rapid improvement of the signal intensity abnormalities was observed [77].

AIDS-associated myelopathy

Vacuolar myelopathy (VM), also known as AIDS-associated myelopathy, is pathologically characterized by vacuolization in the spinal cord with predominantly lateral and posterior column

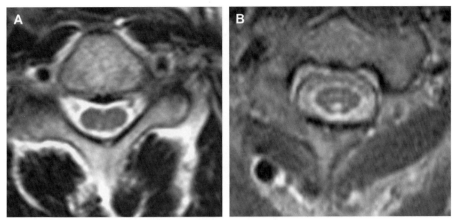

Fig. 13. Subacute combined degeneration in two patients who have gastric cancer and vitamin B12 deficiency. (*A, B*) High-signal-intensity lesions are located in the dorsal aspect of the spinal cord on axial T2-weighted MR images. The cord is not swollen. No enhancement was present on postcontrast images (not shown).

involvement. Edematous swelling within myelin sheaths in the absence of demyelination and in-flammation are pathologic hallmarks of VM [78]. The gross examination of the spinal cord is gener-ally normal unless the disorder is advanced [78]. The frequency of VM reported in the literature ranges from 1% to 55% of patients who have

AIDS [78,79]. In the series by Petito and colleagues [78], 20 of 89 consecutive autopsies of patients who had AIDS showed changes consistent with VM. In-tranuclear viral inclusions in the spinal cord can be seen in only 6% of patients.

Disturbances in vitamin B12 metabolism may play a role in the pathogenesis of VM [80]. The

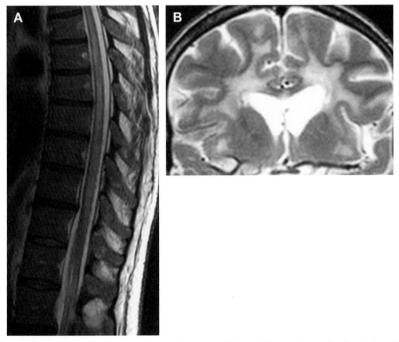

Fig. 14. Vacuolar myelopathy and HIV encephalopathy in an HIV-positive patient who had a low CD4 count and a high viral load level. (*A*) Sagittal T2-weighted MR image showing a high–T2-signal-intensity abnormality in the thoracic spinal cord, extending over multiple segments, without cord swelling. No enhancement was present on postcontrast images (not shown). The findings are nonspecific but are consistent with vacuolar myelopathy in this HIV-positive patient. (*B*) Bilateral high-signal-intensity abnormalities in the frontal white matter are demon-strated on coronal T2-WI MR images, representing HIV encephalopathy.

middle and lower thoracic regions are the most commonly involved areas of the spinal cord [81]. The postmortem pathology in 20 spinal cords of HIV-infected patients who had VM was quantified in one study [82]. Based on the results of the quantitative evaluation, the authors concluded that VM seems to start in the mid-low thoracic cord, with increasing rostral involvement as the disease progresses [82]. The clinical picture of VM includes spastic-ataxic paraparesis, sensory abnormalities in the lower extremities, impotence, and neurogenic bladder [83]. The symptoms usually evolve over several weeks or months and commonly parallel the development of dementia [80]. Recently, an unusual case of VM was described in the literature in an HIV-positive patient who had recurrent clinical symptoms. There were the MR imaging changes typically associated with VM but with a preserved CD4 T-cell count when symptoms occurred for the first time [84]. The characteristic MR imaging findings include bilateral, symmetric, high T2 signal intensity located in the dorsal columns of the spinal cord and extending over multiple segments (Fig. 14) [85,86]. In one study with 55 AIDS patients who had spinal signs and symptoms, two patients were diagnosed with presumed VM [86]. High-signal-intensity abnormalities extending to multiple segments were observed in the cervical spinal cord on T2-WI in both patients. Contrast enhancement was not seen. In another published case of VM, contrast enhancement was also not present [85]. HIV-associated myelitis is less common than VM and usually presents as transverse myelitis. In two cases of presumed HIV myelitis, multifocal, high-signal-intensity abnormalities were described in the lateral and dorsal parts of the cord [86]. Enhancing intramedullary lesions have also been described.

Spinal cord infections

Bacterial myelitis and spinal cord abscess

Staphylococcus aureus and *Streptococcus* are the most common bacterial organisms to invade the spinal cord. Abscess formation in the spinal cord is rare, and hematologic spread is the most common source of infection. Bacterial abscesses have been postulated to occur only in a setting of systemic bacteremia [87]. The contiguous spread of infection through a congenital dermal sinus may be a mechanism in children [88]. The thoracic spine is the most commonly involved part of the cord, with clinical signs and symptoms depending on the location of the lesion [89]. Patients usually present with motor and sensory neurologic deficits and back or radicular pain (60%). Fever is present in 40% of cases. The erythrocyte sedimentation rate tends to be elevated in all patients regardless of clinical findings [89]. CSF cultures are usually sterile. Development of an abscess in the spinal cord may have a phasic course from an early stage of infectious myelitis and from a late stage of myelitis to the final stage of intramedullary cord abscess formation [90]. High signal on T2-weighted MR images with poorly defined enhancement are the typical MR imaging findings in the early stages. Clearly defined peripheral enhancement with surrounding edema is present in the late stage of myelitis. The earliest well defined enhancement was observed 7 days after the onset of symptoms [90]; this is thought to represent the beginning of abscess formation within the spinal cord. In one published report, a case of staphylococcal myelitis of the cervical spinal cord presented as a homogeneously enhancing lesion without cavitation [91]. Because the patient improved clinically and radiologically after antibiotic treatment, the authors postulated that the imaging findings represented early bacterial myelitis resembling pathologically early cerebritis.

Syphilitic myelitis is a rare manifestation of neurosyphilis [92]. High signal abnormality on T2-weighted images, with enhancement predominantly on the surface of the cord, has been described in a few cases of proven syphilitic myelitis

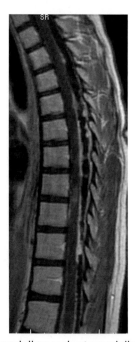

Fig. 15. Intramedullary and extramedullary-intradural tuberculous infection. On a sagittal postcontrast T1-weighted MR image, marked nodular leptomeningeal enhancement is demonstrated. An enhancing lesion is observed in the spinal cord, representing intramedullary tuberculoma.

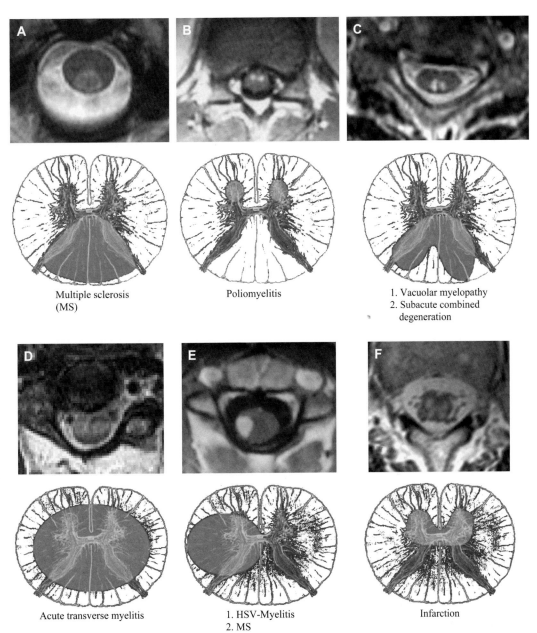

Fig. 16. Differential diagnoses of intramedullary lesions based on their location at the cross-sectional area of the cord. (*A*) MS: Dorsally located wedge-shaped lesion involving less then two thirds of the cross-sectional area of the spinal cord seen on axial T2-Wi MR image. (*B*) Poliomyelitis: Bilateral enhancing anterior nerve roots demonstrated on postcontrast T1-Wi MR image. (*C*) Vacuolar myelopathy: Bilateral, symmetrical, high-signal-intensity abnormality located dorsally in the spinal cord in an HIV-positive patient. DD: Subacute combined degeneration. (*D*) ATM: On axial T2-Wi, a high-signal-intensity lesion involving more than two thirds of cross-sectional area of the spinal cord is observed. (*E*) Herpes-simplex-virus myelitis: Postcontrast T1-Wi axial MR image showing nodular enhancing lesion located in the lateral part of the cervical spinal cord. DD: active MS plaque. (*F*) Spinal cord infarction: Swelling of the anterior parts of the spinal cord is shown on axial T2-Wi MR images, indicating vulnerability of the anterior portions of the spinal cord to ischemia.

[92]. The disappearance of the spinal cord abnormalities suggests the reversible nature of the lesions. In one published case, a high-signal-intensity abnormality was present in the entire spinal cord [92]. Because the clinical and imaging findings are nonspecific, this potentially treatable entity should be included in the differential diagnosis of ATM.

Tuberculosis

Although reports of tuberculosis from developing countries and among HIV-positive patients have increased, intramedullary spinal tuberculosis infection is rare. Intramedullary tuberculomas are seen in 0.002% of the cases of tuberculosis and in 0.2% of the cases of CNS tuberculosis [93], with the ratios of intracranial to intraspinal tuberculomas at 20:1 and 42:1, respectively [94]. MR imaging is the method of choice in detecting spinal cord tuberculoma (Fig. 15). Fusiform swelling of the cord was noted in six of seven cases of intramedullary tuberculoma, with iso- or hyperintensity on T1-WI images [95]. On T2-WI images, a central hypointensity with surrounding hyperintense edema is usually present, a finding suggestive for tuberculoma. A hyperintense center on T2-WI can be present due to the lesser degree of caseation and liquefaction. Solid or ring-like enhancement is usually present on postcontrast images. A case of intramedullary tuberculoma of the thoracic spinal cord was recently reported [96]. MR imaging showed a ring-enhancing mass with perifocal edema within the cord [96]. Tuberculous involvement of the subdural and intramedullary compartment is uncommon; however, a case of a combined subdural spinal tuberculous empyema and intramedullary tuberculoma in an HIV-positive patient has been described [97]. A lentiform lesion with rim enhancement at the T2 level was seen in the cord on postcontrast MR images. In addition, an enhancing subdural collection was present from C5 to further down along the complete thoracic spine, with compression of the spinal cord.

Toxoplasmosis

Spinal cord *Toxoplasma gondii* infection occurs rarely in patients who have AIDS and is associated with coexisting cerebral infection. In one series, 7.3% of 55 patients who had AIDS had spinal cord toxoplasmosis [86]. In a majority of the published reports, an enhancing mass was described in the cord, with low signal intensity on T1-WI and high signal intensity on T2-weighted MR images [86,98–102]. In one patient who had hemophilia-associated AIDS, no abnormalities were present on T1- and T2-weighted MR images, whereas a homogeneously enhancing lesion was detected in the conus without enlargement of the cord on postcontrast images [103].

Summary

Over the past decade, researchers and clinicians have gained new insights into the core of demyelinating diseases of the spinal cord, and much progress has been made in the management of these diseases. Although we are starting to uncover some of the structural and physiologic substrates of demyelination of the CNS, we are far from understanding what causes many of these demyelinating disorders and how to prevent their progression. With further development of new techniques, such as DTI and more potent MR units, spinal cord diseases may be distinguished from each other, and effective therapeutic strategies may be initiated before any cord damage occurs (Fig. 16).

References

[1] Kappos L, Kuhle J, Gass A, et al. Alternatives to current disease-modifying treatment in MS: what do we need and what can we expect in the future? J Neurol 2004;251:57–64.

[2] Ikuta F, Zimmerman HM. Distribution of plaques in seventy autopsy cases of multiple sclerosis in the United States. Neurology 1976;26:26–8.

[3] Toussaint D, Perier O, Verstappen A, et al. Clinicopathological study of the visual pathways, eyes, and cerebral hemispheres in 32 cases of disseminated sclerosis. J Clin Neuroophthalmol 1983;3:211–20.

[4] Carswell R. Pathological anatomy: illustrations of the elementary forms of disease. London: Longman; 1838.

[5] Cruveilhier J. Anatomie pathologique du corps humain; descriptions avec figures lithographiees et calories: des diverses alterations morbides dont le corps humain est susceptible. Paris: Baillier; 1841.

[6] Lycklama G, Thompson A, Filippi M, et al. Spinal cord MRI in multiple sclerosis. Lancet Neurol 2003;2:555–62.

[7] Tench CR, Morgan PS, Jaspan T, et al. Spinal cord imaging in multiple sclerosis. J Neuroimaging 2005;15:94S–102S.

[8] Thielen KR, Miller GM. Multiple sclerosis of the spinal cord: magnetic resonance appearance. J Comput Assist Tomogr 1996;20(3):434–8.

[9] Tartaglino LM, Friedman DP, Flanders AE, et al. Multiple sclerosis in the spinal cord: MR appearance and correlation with clinical parameters. Radiology 1995;195(3):725–32.

[10] Fazekas F, Barkhof F, Filippi M, et al. The contribution of magnetic resonance imaging to the diagnosis of multiple sclerosis. Neurology 1999;53:448–56.

[11] McDonald WI, Compston A, Edan G, et al. Recommended diagnostic criteria for multiple sclerosis: guidelines from the international panel on the diagnosis of multiple sclerosis. Ann Neurol 2001;50:121–7.

[12] Bachmann S, Kesselring J. Multiple sclerosis and infectious childhood diseases. Neuroepidemiology 1998;17(3):154–60.

[13] Dietmann JL, Thibaut-Menard A, Warter JM, et al. MRI in multiple sclerosis of the spinal

cord: evaluation of fast short-tan inversion-recovery and spin-echo sequences. Neuroradiology 2000;42:810–3.

[14] Bot JCJ, Blezer ELA, Kamphorst W, et al. The spinal cord in multiple sclerosis: relationship of high-spatial-resolution quantitative MR imaging findings to histopathological results. Radiology 2004;233:531–40.

[15] Gass A, Filippi M, Rodegher ME, et al. Characteristics of chronic MS lesions in the cerebrum, brainstem, spinal cord, and optic nerve on T1-weighted MRI. Neurology 1998;50:548–50.

[16] Evangelou N, DeLuca GC, Owens T, et al. Pathological study of spinal cord atrophy in multiple sclerosis suggests limited role of local lesions. Brain 2005;128:29–34.

[17] Liu C, Edwards S, Gong Q, et al. Three dimensional MRI estimates of brain and spinal cord atrophy in multiple sclerosis. J Neurol Neurosurg Psychiatry 1999;66(3):323–30.

[18] Bergers E, Bot JCJ, de Groot CJA, et al. Axonal damage in spinal cord of MS patients occurs largely independently of T2 MRI lesions. Neurology 2002;59:1766–71.

[19] Rovaris M, Bozzali M, Santuccio G, et al. Relative contributions of brain and cervical cord pathology to multiple sclerosis disability: a study with magnetisation transfer ratio histogram analysis. J Neurol Neurosurg Psychiatry 2000; 69:723–7.

[20] Ganter P, Prince C, Esiri MM. Spinal cord axonal loss in multiple sclerosis: a post-mortem study. Neuropathol Appl Neurobiol 1999; 25(6):459–67.

[21] Kornek B, Storch MK, Weissert R, et al. Multiple sclerosis and chronic autoimmune encephalomyelitis: a comparative quantitative study of axonal injury in active, inactive, and remyelinated lesions. Am J Pathol 2000;157(1):267–76.

[22] Hittmair K, Mallek R, Prayer D, et al. Spinal cord lesions in patients with multiple sclerosis: comparison of MR pulse sequences. AJNR Am J Neuroradiol 1996;17:1555–65.

[23] Rocca MA, Mastronardo G, Horsfield MA, et al. Comparison of three MR sequences for the detection of cervical cord lesions in patients with multiple sclerosis. AJNR Am J Neuroradiol 1999;244:119–24.

[24] Bot JCJ, Barkhof F, Lyclama a Nijeholt G, et al. Differentiation of multiple sclerosis from other inflammatory disorders and cerebrovascular disease: value of spinal MR imaging. Radiology 2002;233:46–56.

[25] Paty DW, Oger JJ, Kastrukoff LF, et al. MRI in the diagnosis of MS: a prospective study with comparison of clinical evaluation, evoked potentials, oligoclonal banding, and CT. Neurology 1988;38:180–5.

[26] Fazekas F, Offenbacher H, Fuchs S, et al. Criteria for an increased specificity of MRI interpretation in elderly subjects with suspected multiple sclerosis. Neurology 1988;38:1822–5.

[27] Barkhof F, Filippi M, Miller DH, et al. Comparison of MRI criteria at first presentation to predict conversion to clinically definite multiple sclerosis. Brain 1997;120:2059–69.

[28] Bammer R. Basic principles of diffusion-weighted imaging. Eur J Radiol 2003;43: 169–84.

[29] Thurnher MM, Bammer R. Diffusion-weighted MR imaging (DWI) in spinal cord ischemia. Neuroradiology 2006;48(11):795–801.

[30] Clark CA, Werring DJ, Miller DH. Diffusion imaging of the spinal cord in vivo: estimation of the principal diffusivities and application to multiple sclerosis. Magn Reson Med 2000;43: 133–8.

[31] Larsson HBW, Thomsen C, Fredriksen J, et al. In vivo magnetic resonance diffusion measurements in the brain of patients with multiple sclerosis. Magn Reson Imaging 1992;10:7–12.

[32] Christensen P, Gideon P, Thomsen C, et al. Increased water self-diffusion in chronic plaques and in apparently normal white matter in patients with multiple sclerosis. Acta Neurol Scand 1993;87:195–7.

[33] Werring DJ, Clark CA, Barker GJ, et al. Diffusion tensor imaging of lesions and normal appearing white matter in multiple sclerosis. Neurology 1999;52:1626–32.

[34] Lycklama a Nijeholt GJ, Bergers E, Kamphorst W, et al. Post-mortem high-resolution MRI of the spinal cord in multiple sclerosis: a correlative study with conventional MRI, histopathology and clinical phenotype. Brain 2001;124:154–66.

[35] Valsasina P, Rocca MA, Agosta F, et al. Mean diffusivity and fractional anisotropy histogram analysis of the cervical cord in MS patients. Neuroimage 2005;26:822–8.

[36] Hasseltine SM, Law M, Babb J, et al. Diffusion tensor imaging in multiple sclerosis: assessment of regional differences in the axial plane within normal-appearing cervical spinal cord. AJNR Am J Neuroradiol 2006;27(6):1189–93.

[37] Agosta F, Benedetti B, Rocca MA, et al. Quantification of cervical cord pathology in primary progressive MS using diffusion tensor MRI. Neurology 2005;22:631–5.

[38] Hickmann SJ, Hadjiprocopis A, Coulon O, et al. Cervical spinal cord MTR histogram analysis in multiple sclerosis using 3D acquisition and a B-spline active surface segmentation technique. Magn Reson Imaging 2004;22:891–5.

[39] Bozalli M, Rocca MA, Iannucci G, et al. Magnetization-transfer histogram analysis of the cervical cord in patients with multiple sclerosis. AJNR Am J Neuroradiol 1999;20:1803–8.

[40] Filippi M, Bozzali M, Horsfield MA, et al. A conventional and magnetization transfer MRI study of the cervical spinal cord in patients with MS. Neurology 2000;54:207–13.

[41] Devic E. Myelite subaiguë compliquée de névrite optique. Bull Med 1894;8:1033–4.

[42] Mandler RN, Gambarelli D, Gayraud D, et al. Devic's neuromyelitis optica: a clinicopathological study of 8 patients. Ann Neurol 1993;34:162–8.

[43] Filippi M, Rocca MA. MR imaging of Devic's neuromyelitis optica. Neurol Sci 2004;25:S371–3.

[44] Wingerchuk DM, Weinshenker BG. Neuromyelitis optica: clinical predictors of a relapsing course and survival. Neurology 2003;60:848–53.

[45] Ghezzi A, Bergamaschi R, Martinelli V, et al. Clinical characteristics, course and prognosis of relapsing Devic's neuromyelitis optica. J neurol 2004;251:47–52.

[46] Fardet L, Genereau T, Mikaeloff Y, et al. Devic's neuromyelitis optica: study of nine cases. Acta Neurol Scand 2003;108:193–200.

[47] Tashiro K, Ito K, Maruo Y, et al. MR imaging in spinal cord in Devic disease. J Comput Assist Tomogr 1987;11:516–7.

[48] Barkhof F, Scheltens P, Valk J, et al. Serial quantitative MR assessment of optic neuritis in a case of neuromyelitis optica, using Gadolinium-"enhanced" STIR imaging. Neuroradiology 1991;33:70–1.

[49] Lennon VA, Wingerchik DM, Kryzer TJ, et al. A serum autoantibody marker of neuromyelitis optica: distinction from multiple sclerosis. Lancet 2004;364(9451):2106–12.

[50] Rocca MA, Agosta F, Mezzapesa DM, et al. Magnetization transfer and diffusion tensor MRI show gray matter damage in neuromyelitis optica. Neurology 2004;10(62):476–8.

[51] Bastian HC. Special diseases of the spinal cord. In: Quain R, editor. A dictionary of medicine: including general pathology, general therapeutics, hygiene, and the diseases peculiar to women and children. London: Longmans, Green; 1882. p. 1479–83.

[52] Suchett-Kaye AL. Acute transverse myelitis complicating pneumonia. Lancet 1948;255:417.

[53] Krishnan C, Kaplin AI, Pardo CA, et al. Demyelinating disorders: update on transverse myelitis. Curr Neurol Neurosci Rep 2006;6(3):236–43.

[54] Kerr DA, Ayetey H. Immunopathogenesis of acute transverse myelitis. Curr Opin Neurol 2002;15:339–47.

[55] Larner AJ, Farmer SF. Myelopathy following influenza vaccination in inflammatory CNS disorder treated with chronic immunosuppression. Eur J Neurol 2000;7:731–3.

[56] Bakshi R, Mazziotta JC. Acute transverse myelitis after influenza vaccination: magnetic resonance imaging findings. J Neuroimaging 1996;6(4):248–50.

[57] De Seze J, Lanctin C, Lebrun C, et al. Idiopathic acute transverse myelitis: application of the recent diagnostic criteria. Neurology 2005;65:1950–3.

[58] Transverse Myelitis Consortium Working Group (TMCWG). Proposed diagnostic criteria and nosology of acute transverse myelitis. Neurology 2002;59:499–505.

[59] Choi KH, Lee KS, Chung SO, et al. Idiopathic transverse myelitis: MR characteristics. AJNR Am J Neuroradiol 1996;17:1151–60.

[60] Kim KK. Idiopathic reccurent transverse myelitis. Arch Neurol 2003;60:1290–4.

[61] Brinar VV, Habek M, Brinar M, et al. The differential diagnosis of acute transverse myelitis. Clin Neurol Neurosurg 2006;108:278–83.

[62] Holtas S, Basibüyük N, Fredriksson K. MRI in acute transverse myelopathy. Neuroradiology 1993;35:221–6.

[63] Scotti G, Gerevini S. Diagnosis and differential diagnosis of acute transverse myelopathy: the role of neuroradiological investigations and review of the literature. Neurol Sci 2001;22(2):S69–73.

[64] Pittock SJ, Lucchinetti CF. Inflammatory transverse myelitis: evolving concepts. Current Opin Neurol 2006;19:362–8.

[65] Renoux J, Facon D, Fillard P, et al. MR diffusion tensor imaging and fiber tracking in inflammatory diseases of the spinal cord. AJNR Am J Neuroradiol 2006;27:1947–51.

[66] Cree BA, Wingerchuk DM. Acute transverse myelitis: is the "idiopathic" form vanishing? Neurology 2005;65(12):1857–8.

[67] Schwarz S, Mohr A, Knauth M, et al. Acute disseminated encephalomyelitis: a follow-up study of 40 adult patients. Neurology 2001;56:1313–8.

[68] Poser CM. Magnetic resonance imaging in asymptomatic disseminated vasculinomyelopathy. J Neurol Sci 1989;94:69–77.

[69] Spieker S, Petersen D, Rolfs A, et al. Acute disseminated encephalomyelitis following Pontiac fever. Eur Neurol 1998;40:169–72.

[70] Singh S, Prabhakar S, Korah IP, et al. Acute disseminated encephalomyelitis and multiple sclerosis: magnetic resonance imaging differentiation. Australas Radiol 2000;44:404–11.

[71] Khong PL, Ho HK, Cheng PW, et al. Childhood acute disseminated encephalomyelitis: the role of brain and spinal cord MRI. Pediatr Radiol 2002;32:59–66.

[72] Rust RS. Multiple sclerosis, acute disseminated encephalomyelitis, and related conditions. Semin Pediatr Neurol 2000;7(2):66–90.

[73] Inglese M, Salvi F, Iannucco G, et al. Magnetization transfer and diffusion tensor MR imaging of acute disseminated encephalomyelitis. AJNR Am J Neuroradiol 2002;23:267–72.

[74] Hemmer B, Glocker FX, Schumacher M, et al. Subacute combined degeneration: clinical, electrophysiological, and magnetic resonance imaging findings. J Neurol Neurosurg Psychiatry 1998;65:822–7.

[75] Yamada K, Shier DA, Tanaka H, et al. A case of subacute combined degeneration: MRI findings. Neuroradiology 1998;40:398–400.

[76] Karantanas AH, Markonis A, Bisbiyiannis G. Subacute combined degeneration of the spinal cord with involvement of the anterior columns: a new MRI finding. Neuroradiology 2000;42: 115–7.

[77] Berlit P, Ringelstein A, Liebig T. Spinal MRI precedes clinical improvement in subacute combined degeneration with B12 deficiency. Neurology 2004;63:592–3.

[78] Petito CK, Navia BA, Cho ES, et al. Vacuolar myelopathy pathologically resembling subacute combined degeneration in patients with the acquired immunodeficiency syndrome. N Engl J Med 1985;312:874–9.

[79] Henin D, Smith TW, De Girolami U, et al. Neuropathology of the spinal cord in the acquired immunodeficiency syndrome. Hum Pathol 1992; 23:1106–14.

[80] McArthur JC, Brew BJ, Nath A. Neurological complications of HIV infection. Lancet Neurol 2005;4:543–55.

[81] Berger JR, Sabet A. Infectious myelopathies. Semin Neurol 2002;22(2):133–42.

[82] Tan SV, Guiloff RJ, Scaravilli F. AIDS-associated vacuolar myelopathy: a morphometric study. Brain 1995;118:1247–61.

[83] Di Rocco A, Bottiglieri T, Werner P, et al. Abnormal cobalamin-dependent transmethylation in AIDS-associated myelopathy. Neurology 2002; 58:730–5.

[84] Anneken K, Fischera M, Evers S, et al. Recurrent vacuolar myelopathy in HIV infection. J Infect 2006;52:181–3.

[85] Sartoretti-Schefer S, Blattler T, Wichmann W. Spinal MRI in vacuolar myelopathy, and correlation with histopathological findings. Neuroradiology 1997;39:865–9.

[86] Thurnher MM, Post MJD, Jinkins R. MRI of infections and neoplasms of the spine and spinal cord in 55 patients with AIDS. Neuroradiology 2000;42:551–63.

[87] Babu R, Jafar JJ, Huang PP, et al. Intramedullary cord abscesses associated with spinal cord ependymoma. Neurosurgery 1992;30:121–4.

[88] Chan CT, Gold WL. Intramedullary abscess of the spinal cord in the antibiotic era: clinical features, microbial etiologies, trends in pathogenesis, and outcomes. Clin Infect Dis 1998;27: 619–26.

[89] Candon E, Frerebeau P. Bacterial abscesses of the spinal cord: review of the literature (73 cases). Rev Neurol 1994;150:370–6.

[90] Murphy KJ, Brunberg JA, Quint DJ, et al. Spinal cord infection: myelitis and abscess formation. AJNR Am J Neuroradiol 1988;19:341–8.

[91] Friess HM, Wasenko JJ. MR of staphylococcal myelitis of the cervical spinal cord. AJNR Am J Neuroradiol 1997;18:455–8.

[92] Tsui EYK, Ng SH, Chow L, et al. Syphilitic myelitis with diffuse spinal cord abnormality on MR imaging. Eur Radiol 2002;12:2973–6.

[93] Citow JS, Ammirati M. Intramedullary tuberculoma of the spinal cord: case report. Neurosurgery 1994;35:327–30.

[94] Jinkins JR, Gupta R, Chang KH, et al. MR imaging of central nervous system tuberculosis. Radiol Clin North Am 1995;33(4):771–86.

[95] Parmar H, Shah J, Patkar D, et al. Intramedullary tuberculomas: MR findings in seven patients. Acta Radiol 2000;41:572–7.

[96] Torii H, Takahashi T, Shimizu H, et al. Intramedullary spinal tuberculoma: case report. Neurol Med Chir (Tokyo) 2004;44:266–8.

[97] Alessi G, Lemmerling M, Nathoo N. Combined spinal subdural tuberculous empyema and intramedullary tuberculoma in an HIV-positive patient. Eur Radiol 2003;13:1899–901.

[98] Fairley CK, Wodak J, Benson E. Spinal cord toxoplasmosis in a patient with human immunodeficiency virus infection. Int J STD AIDS 1992;3:366–8.

[99] Harris TM, Smith RR, Bognanno JR, et al. Toxoplasmic myelitis in AIDS: gadolinium-enhanced MR. J Comput Assist Tomogr 1990;14:809–11.

[100] Mehren M, Burns PJ, Mamani F, et al. Toxoplasmic myelitis mimicking intramedullary spinal cord tumor. Neurology 1988;38:1648–50.

[101] Poon TP, Tchertkoff V, Pares F, et al. Spinal cord toxoplasma lesion in AIDS: MR findings. J Comput Assist Tomogr 1992;16:817–9.

[102] Resnick DK, Comey CH, Welch WC, et al. Isolated toxoplasmosis of the thoracic spinal cord in a patient with acquired immunodeficiency syndrome. J Neurosurg 1995;82:493–6.

[103] Kayser K, Campbell R, Sartorious C, et al. Toxoplasmosis of the conus medullaris in a patient with hemophilia A-associated AIDS. J Neurosurg 1990;73:951–3.

NEUROIMAGING
CLINICS
OF NORTH AMERICA

Neuroimag Clin N Am 17 (2007) 57–72

Imaging in Spinal Vascular Disease

Timo Krings, MD, PhD[a,b,c,]*, Pierre L. Lasjaunias, MD, PhD[b],
Franz J. Hans, MD[c], Michael Mull, MD[a], Robbert J. Nijenhuis, MD[d],
Hortensia Alvarez, MD[b], Walter H. Backes, PhD[d],
Marcus H.T. Reinges, MD[c], Georges Rodesch, MD, PhD[b],
Joachim M. Gilsbach, MD, PhD[c], Armin K. Thron, MD, PhD[a]

- Anatomy
- Spinal cord ischemia
- Spinal vascular malformations
- Dural arteriovenous fistulae
- Spinal cord arteriovenous malformations
- Cavernomas
- Summary
- References

Spinal vascular diseases are a rare entity (1%–2%) within vascular neurologic pathologic conditions. Their clinical diagnosis rests mainly on MRI, although for a thorough understanding of the diseases involved and the therapeutic strategy, digital subtraction angiography (DSA) still is necessary. In this article we first discuss the normal vascular anatomy of the spine. Second, we describe causes, symptoms, and imaging findings of spinal cord ischemia. Third, we discuss spinal vascular malformations that typically lead to progressive spinal cord symptoms and myelopathy if not properly treated. Depending on the type of spinal vascular disease, initial symptoms may vary between acute or chronic onset. Pathophysiologic mechanisms include arterial ischemia, intramedullary or subarachnoidal hemorrhages, or subacute venous congestion leading to progressive myelopathy. The space-occupying nature of some of these lesions and a circulatory "steal" phenomenon are additional possible pathophysiologic mechanisms. Although acute manifestations of spinal vascular malformations are typically diagnosed early in the course of the disease, the subacute venous congestion might lead to unspecific neurologic symptoms, which in turn delay proper diagnosis. The aim of this article is to review the imaging features, clinical symptomatology, and potential therapeutic approaches of spinal vascular malformations and remind the neuroradiologists and referring physicians that the diagnosis and subsequent treatment of these treatable causes of severe and otherwise progressive neurologic deficits still remain a challenge.

Anatomy

To interpret MRI and DSA findings of spinal vascular diseases, it is necessary to be aware of the normal arterial supply and venous drainage of the spine and spinal cord. Segmental arteries supply the

[a] Department of Neuroradiology, University Hospital Aachen, Pauwelsstrasse 30, 52057 Aachen, Germany
[b] Service de Neuroradiologie Diagnostique et Thérapeutique, Hôpital de Bicetre, 78 Rue du General Leclerc, 94275 Le Kremlin-Bicetre CEDEX, France
[c] Department of Neurosurgery, University Hospital Aachen, Pauwelsstrasse 30, 52057 Aachen, Germany
[d] Department of Radiology, University Hospital Maastricht, p. Debyelaan 25, 6202 AZ Maastricht, The Netherlands
* Corresponding author. Department of Neuroradiology, University Hospital, University of Technology, Aachen, Pauwelsstrasse 30, 52057 Aachen, Germany.
E-mail address: tkrings@ukaachen.de (T. Krings).

doi:10.1016/j.nic.2007.01.001

spine, including the vertebral bodies, paraspinal muscles, dura, nerve roots, and the spinal cord with blood. Radicular arteries are the first branches of the dorsal division of the segmental arteries. The bony spine is supplied by anterior and posterior central arteries that come directly from the segmental and radicular arteries [1]. A spinal radicular branch that supplies the dura and nerve root as a radiculomeningeal artery is present at each segment. From these radicular arteries, radiculomedullary and radiculopial arteries might branch, following the anterior or posterior nerve root to reach the anterior or posterior surface of the cord, where they form the anterior or posterior spinal artery [2].

In adult patients, not all lumbar or intercostal arteries have a radiculomedullary feeder, and their location for a given patient is not predictable. The anterior and posterior spinal arteries constitute a superficial longitudinal anastomosing system [3]. The anterior spinal artery travels along the anterior sulcus and typically originates from the two vertebral arteries, whereas the typically paired posterolateral spinal arteries originate from the preatlantal part of the vertebral artery or from the posteroinferior cerebellar artery. These three arteries run from the cervical spine to the conus medullaris but are not capable of feeding the entire spinal cord. Instead, they are reinforced from the radiculomedullary arteries that derive from various (and unpredictable) segmental levels by anterior and posterolateral radiculomedullary arteries [4]. The most well known of the anterior radiculomedullary arteries is the artery radiculomedullaris magna (ie, the Adamkiewicz artery). The anterior radiculomedullary arteries branch in a typical way to reach the spinal cord. The ascending branch continues along the direction of the radicular artery in the midline of the anterior surface. The descending branch, being the larger one at thoracolumbar levels, forms a hairpin curve as soon as it reaches the midline at the entrance of the anterior fissure [2].

The intrinsic network of the spinal cord arteries can be divided into central or sulcal arteries from the anterior spinal artery and into the rami perforantes of the vasacorona that supplies the periphery of the spinal cord and is derived from the anterior and paired posterolateral arteries [3].

The spinal cord is protected against ischemia by longitudinal and transverse anastomoses. Extradurally, interconnections between segmental arteries can compensate for a proximal occlusion of a radicular artery, whereas intradurally, the anterior and posterior spinal arteries represent a system of longitudinal anastomoses that is reinforced from different levels. The posterior and anterior arterial systems are interconnected at the level of the cone via the "basket" anastomosis and via transverse anastomoses of the intrinsic arteries that interconnect by the pial network of the vasacorona [3]. Spinal infarctions are highly variable, and predictable vascular territories as present in the brain do not exist.

The venous drainage of the cord is via radially symmetric intrinsic spinal cord veins and small superficial pial veins that open into the superficial longitudinal median anastomosing spinal cord veins. These veins more or less follow the arteries (ie, the anterior and posterior median spinal vein) but have many anastomoses (including transmedullary anastomoses) that create a network with commonly more than one anterior and posterior vein [4]. They may also use the roots as a vehicle to reach the epidural plexus and the extraspinal veins and plexus with a reflux-impeding mechanism within the dura mater [5]. It is important to note that the transition of a median vein into a radicular vein shows the same hairpin shape as the artery. At the superior cervical part, they can run through the occipital foramen to connect to the vertebral plexus or the inferior dural sinus. Drainage of blood from the spine occurs through the valveless internal and external venous vertebral plexus, which is connected to the azygos and hemiazygos venous systems [1].

Spinal cord ischemia

Compared with brain ischemia, spinal cord infarction is exceedingly rare and caused by more diverse etiologies [1]. This rarity is mainly caused by the multiple anastomoses of the spinal cord, which supply arteries. Spinal cord supplying arteries are—for unknown reasons—not significantly affected by atherosclerotic vessel wall changes. Causes for acute arterial ischemia include surgery for aortoiliac occlusive disease [6], dissection of the aorta, vasculitis, fibrocartilaginous embolism [7], Caisson disease, lumbar artery compression [8], cardiac arrest and systemic hypotension, thrombosis/embolism, coagulopathies, and toxic effects of contrast medium. Acute ischemia has an acute onset; transverse cord symptoms and radicular pain are common initial complaints. Symptoms may include nerve root deficits or sphincter weakness. Typical clinical symptoms (ie, an anterior spinal artery syndrome) are the exception rather than the rule because of the high variability of spinal cord vascular supply. Common sites of spinal cord infarction are the thoracolumbar enlargement and the conus medullaris [1].

MRI is the diagnostic modality of choice; however, in the early phase it can show negative results on routine sequences, because only 50% of patients show an early demarcation of T2 hyperintensity of the spine within the first 24 hours. The role of MRI in the acute phase is to rule out other lesions that might go along with an acute nontraumatic transverse spinal lesion. On T2-weighted images, a pencil-shaped T2 hyperintensity is visible predominantly in the anterior part of the cord, typically sparing the outer rim of the cord (Figs. 1 and 2) [9]. In few studies, spinal diffusion–weighted images were performed in spinal cord infarction [10–12]. These studies found an area of reduced diffusion after 8 hours (Fig. 3).

Moderate swelling is generally present in the acute stage followed by contrast enhancement of the cord and the cauda equina in the subacute stage (typically after 5 days) (Fig. 4). Contrast enhancement may persist for up to 3 weeks after onset [1]. Abnormal signal or evolution of signal abnormalities within the vertebral body caused by associated vertebral body infarction often is encountered (Fig. 5) [13]. The field of view should be large enough to rule out aortic dissection.

Spinal vascular malformations

Multiple different classification schemes have been proposed for spinal vascular malformations. Recently, the Bicetre group classified spinal cord arteriovenous malformations (AVMs) into three main groups [14]. The first group includes genetic hereditary lesions that are caused by a genetic disorder affecting the vascular germinal cells. Spinal cord malformations associated to hereditary hemorrhagic telangiectasia fall into this category. The second group includes genetic nonhereditary lesions that share metameric links, such as Cobb syndrome (or spinal AV metameric syndrome), that affect the whole myelomere. Patients typically present with multiple shunts of the spinal cord, the nerve root, bone, paraspinal, subcutaneous, and skin tissues. Klippel-Trenaunay and Parkes-Weber syndromes also belong to this group. The third group includes single lesions that may reflect the incomplete expression of one of the previous mentioned situations and includes spinal cord, nerve root, and lesions of the filum terminale.

For practical therapeutic reasons and because most spinal vascular malformations fall into the last group, we use a classification that is based on the vascular anatomy of the spinal cord and the inborn or acquired nature of the lesion [15]. According to this classification, spinal vascular malformations can be differentiated, similar to vascular malformations of the brain, into true inborn lesions and the acquired lesions, the latter being dural AV fistulae, whereas AVMs and cavernomas constitute inborn lesions of the spine (Table 1) [16]. In contrast to the brain, in which capillary teleangiectases also belong to the inborn lesions, they have not been found in the spine and are not discussed further.

Spinal cord AVMs are like their cerebral counterparts malformations, which are fed by arteries that normally supply the neural tissue (ie, the intrinsic

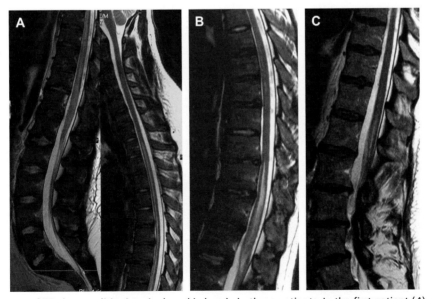

Fig. 1. Spectrum of T2 abnormalities in spinal cord ischemia in three patients. In the first patient (*A*), the hyperintensity extends from the cone to Th1. In the second patient (*B*), the signal abnormalities extend over three segments. In the third patient (*C*), the signal abnormality is confined to the cone. This image demonstrates the large variability of craniocaudal extension of spinal cord ischemia.

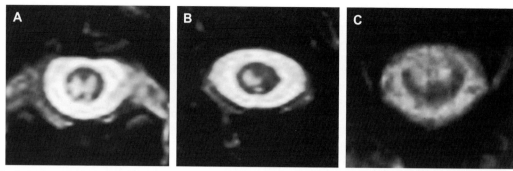

Fig. 2. Spectrum of T2 abnormalities in spinal cord ischemia in three patients. (*A–C*) These images demonstrate the variability in transverse extension of spinal cord ischemia that is caused by anatomic variations of anastomoses of the anterior spinal artery system.

arteries of the spinal cord), whereas spinal cord dural AV fistulae are like their cranial counterparts, the dural AV fistulae, which are fed by radiculomeningeal arteries (similar to meningeal arteries) [16].

Dural arteriovenous fistulae

Spinal dural AV fistulae are the most frequent vascular malformations of the spine and account for 70% of all AV shunts of the spine [16]. They

are presumably acquired lesions; however, the exact etiology is not known. Usually the disease becomes symptomatic in older men (aged 40–60 years) [17]. Most fistulae are located in the thoracolumbar region. The AV shunt is located inside the dura mater close to the spinal nerve root, where the arterial blood from a radiculomeningeal artery (ie, an artery supplying the root and meninges but not necessarily the spinal cord) enters a radicular vein, where the latter passes the dura.

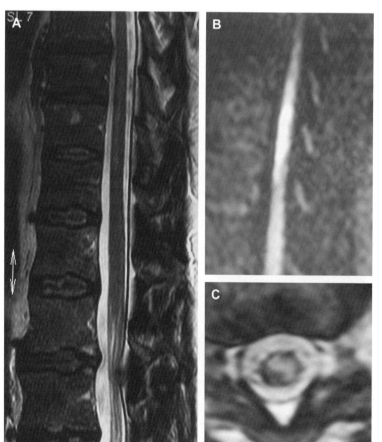

Fig. 3. A 55-year-old man with acute onset of severe stabbing back pain followed by subacute onset of paraplegia. (*A*) Sagittal T2-weighted image 8 hours after onset of symptoms shows a subtle pencil-shaped hyperintensity of the spinal cord. (*B*) On diffusion-weighted sagittal MRI, a large area of diffusion abnormality can be seen indicating spinal cord ischemia. (*C*) On follow-up axial T2-weighted images, a hyperintensity of the central parts of the spinal cord sparing the outer rim can be seen, which indicates spinal cord ischemia in the territory of the anterior spinal artery.

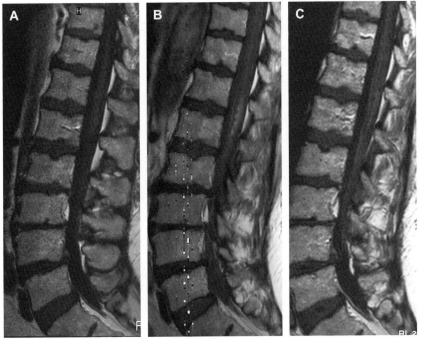

Fig. 4. Evolution of contrast enhancement after spinal cord ischemia. (*A*) Initial postcontrast T1-weighted MRI in a sagittal plane demonstrates no pathologic enhancement, whereas first follow-up MR scan (*B*) (after 10 days) and second follow-up MR examination (*C*) (after 18 days) demonstrate enhancement of the conus and the cauda equina. Contrast enhancement after spinal cord ischemia typically appears after the fifth day, including the conus and the cauda as a sign for disruption of the blood-brain barrier and a reactive hyperemia.

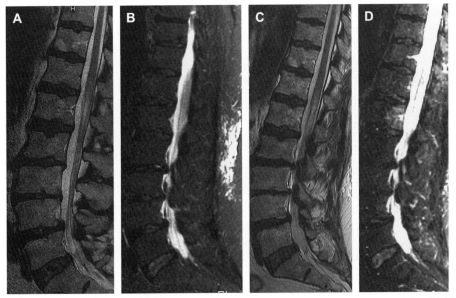

Fig. 5. Evolution of T2 and STIR changes after spinal cord ischemia. Initial T2- (*A*) and STIR-weighted (*B*) images 1 hour after the onset of acute stabbing back pain and paraplegia demonstrate essentially normal findings. T2- (*C*) and STIR-weighted (*D*) images 3 days after the event show the spinal cord ischemia as a hyperintensity of the cone and an associated vertebral body infarction on the STIR-weighted images.

Table 1: Classification of spinal vascular malformations

Type	Etiology	Feeding artery	Draining vein	Pathophysiology	Age of onset (y)	Therapy
AVM						
Perimedullary fistula (types I–III)	Inborn	Radiculomedullary	Intramedullary and superficial spinal cord veins → epidural venous plexus (orthograde)	Intraparenchymal or subarachnoid hemorrhage, chronic venous congestion, space occupation	20–40	Type I: surgery; types II, III: coil or balloon embolization
Glomerular					<20	Particle or glue embolization
Juvenile					<15	Embolization and/or surgery
Cavernoma	Inborn	NA	NA	Hemorrhage and progressive myelopathy	20–60	Surgery
Dural AV fistula	Acquired	Radiculomeningeal	Radicular vein → perimedullary veins (retrograde)	Chronic venous congestion	40–60	Surgery or glue embolization

Abbreviation: NA, not applicable.

The increase in spinal venous pressure diminishes the AV pressure gradient and leads to a decreased drainage of normal spinal veins and venous congestion with intramedullary edema [18,19]. This development leads to chronic hypoxia and progressive myelopathy [20]. Clinical symptomatology of this congestive myelopathy is unspecific and might consist of hypo- and paraesthesias, paraparesis, back pain that might radiate to the lower legs, impotence, and sphincter disturbances. Usually the deficits are slowly progressive; however, an acute onset of the disease and progressive development interrupted by intermediate remissions is also possible [16,21]. Without therapy, this therapy results in irreversible para- or even tetraplegia.

On MRI the combination of cord edema and perimedullary dilated vessels is the characteristic finding and should lead to the diagnosis [21]. On T2-weighted sequences, the cord edema is depicted as a centromedullary, not well-delineated hyperintensity over multiple segments that is often accompanied by a hypointense rim, which most likely represents deoxygenated blood within the dilated capillary vessels surrounding the congestive edema (Figs. 6 and 7) [22]. The cord is swollen and might demonstrate contrast enhancement as a sign for chronic venous congestion (Fig. 8) [23]. In the further course of the disease, the cord atrophies

(Fig. 9). The perimedullary vessels are dilated and coiled and can be observed on T2-weighted images as flow voids. If the shunt volume is small, however, they might only be seen after contrast enhancement. Neither the location of pathologic vessels nor the intramedullary imaging findings seem to be related to the height of the fistula.

Localization of the fistula sometimes can be difficult, leading to lengthy and even multiple catheterization procedures. Noninvasive diagnostic techniques, such as contrast-enhanced MR angiography with relative fast acquisition protocols, have been developed [24–26]. Apart from identifying the segmental level of the fistula, it is necessary to localize the spinal cord–supplying arteries, especially the great anterior radiculomedullary artery (ie, the Adamkiewicz artery). Prior knowledge of the location of the Adamkiewicz artery may prevent neurologic complications when performing therapeutic procedures. To depict and separate the submillimeter-sized spinal cord arteries from the spinal cord veins, a simultaneously high spatial and temporal resolution should be achieved. A large craniocaudal field of view must be used because the location of the fistula is highly variable and cannot be pinpointed to findings previously obtained by conventional MRI.

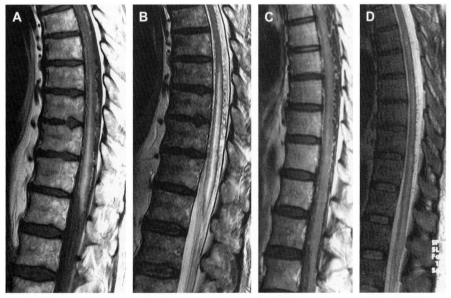

Fig. 6. Spectrum of MRI findings in spinal dural AV fistulae in two patients. (*A–D*) On T1-weighted images after contrast injection (*A, C*), dilated and tortuous perimedullary vessels can be seen, which are visible as pathologic flow voids along the dorsal surface of the spinal cord on T2-weighted images (*B, D*). On sagittal postcontrast T1-weighted MRI (*A*), a contrast enhancement of the conus as a sign for subacute venous infarction can be appreciated. As can be seen from these two patients, the amount of intramedullary edema can be highly variable, ranging from a few segments to the entire cord. Typically, the edema is not well delineated from the cord and comes along with a swelling of the cord.

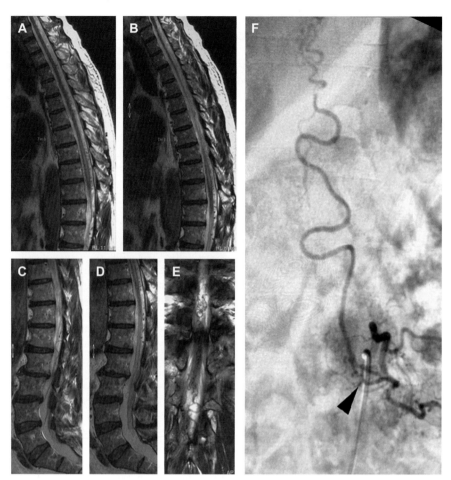

Fig. 7. Spinal dural AV fistula: MRI and DSA. (*A–E*) On T2-weighted images the conus is slightly hyperintense. The most striking findings are the tortuous and dilated perimedullary vessels, which are present as a flow void in these images. The combination of pathologically dilated vessels and edema of the cord is pathognomonic for spinal dural AV fistulae. Angiography, however, is necessary to rule out a small perimedullary fistula and localize the height of the fistula. The arrowhead (*F*) demonstrates the fistulous zone at the level of L3 on the left side.

Recently, contrast-enhanced MR angiography featuring centric K-space filling and a large field of view, validated by DSA, was able to depict the spinal cord arteries and veins. The need for a large field of view to localize the fistula level can be best demonstrated by two recent MR angiography studies, which reported that localization was not always successful in the first MR angiography examination because of a small field of view [25]. The MR angiography approach using a larger field of view has shown promising results (Fig. 10) [26]. The efficacy of this technique for the localization of the fistula must be investigated further, however. Spinal catheter angiography is still necessary to verify the exact height of the fistula and rule out a type I perimedullary fistula, which might have the same imaging appearances on MR angiography.

There are two options in the treatment of spinal dural AV fistulae: surgical occlusion of the intradural vein that receives the blood from the shunt zone—a relatively simple and safe intervention with exception of sacral fistulae [24,25]—or endovascular therapy using glue after superselective catheterization of the feeding radiculomeningeal artery [26,27]. The embolic agent must pass the nidus and reach and occlude the proximal segment of the draining vein to prevent subsequent intradural collateral filling of the fistula. Success rates of endovascular therapy have been reported to vary between 25% and 75% [26,28]. After complete occlusion of the fistula, the progression of the disease can be stopped; however, only two thirds of all patients have a regression of their motor symptomatology, and only one third show an improvement in their

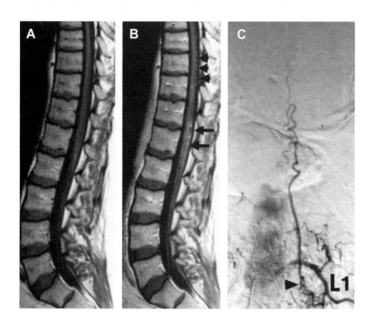

Fig. 8. Spinal dural AV fistula on T1-weighted images before (*A*) and after (*B*) contrast and on DSA (*C*). (*B*) The conus demonstrates slight contrast enhancement as a sign for chronic ischemic changes (*arrows*). Pathologic vessels can be defined easily after contrast enhancement (*arrowheads*). (*C*) On angiography, the fistula was found arising from the radiculomeningeal artery of the L1 segmental artery (*arrowhead* at site of fistulation).

sensory disturbances. Impotence and sphincter disturbances are seldom reversible [29].

Spinal cord arteriovenous malformations

Spinal cord AVMs are fed by radicullomedullary (ie, spinal cord) feeding arteries and drained by spinal cord veins. These high-flow shunts might be intra- or perimedullarily located and can be differentiated according to their transition from artery into vein into fistulous and glomerular AVMs [30]. Glomerular AVMs (which are sometimes called plexiforme or nidus-type AVMs) are the most often encountered spinal cord AVMs, with a nidus resembling that of a brain AVM. This type of malformation usually is located intramedullarily. Superficial nidus compartments can, however, also reach the subarachnoid space. Because of the many anastomoses between the anterior and posterior arterial feeding system of the spine, these AVMs typically have multiple arteries derived from the posterior and anterior systems. Drainage is into dilated spinal cord vessels (Figs. 11–13).

Fistulous AVMs (which are also called AVMs of the perimedullary fistula type or intradural AV fistulae) are direct AV shunts located superficially on the

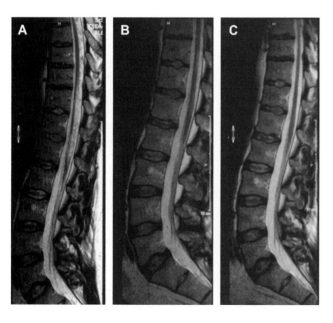

Fig. 9. Atrophy of the spinal cord after occlusion of a long-existing spinal dural AV fistula. (*A, B*) Before obliteration of the fistula, a swollen hyperintense spinal cord can be perceived (*A*), which disappears after obliteration (*B*). (*C*) Twelve months after occlusion of the fistula, the cord edema is absent; however, the cord atrophies because of long-existing chronic venous hypertension.

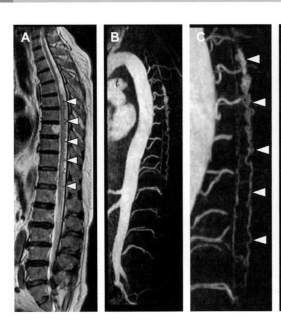

Fig. 10. Advances in time-resolved, contrast-enhanced MR angiography have enabled us to noninvasively detect the area of fistulation in dural AV fistula, as can be demonstrated in this patient with a spinal dural AV fistula at the level of TH7. This technique proves helpful in determining the height of fistulation before selective spinal DSA. (*A*) T2-weighted MRI shows flow voids and cord edema. (*B, C*) Lateral projection of the arterial phase of the contrast-enhanced MR angiography shows pathologic veins present in the arterial phase. Coronal reconstruction of these images (*D*) clearly indicates the level of the shunt, which was confirmed during spinal DSA.

spinal cord and only rarely possess intramedullary compartments [31]. Feeding vessels are radiculomedullary arteries (which differentiates them from the dural AV fistulae, which were discussed previously). Draining veins are superficial perimedullary veins. The arterialized blood sometimes even ascends via the foramen magnum into the posterior fossa. Fistulous AVMs can be subdivided into three types depending on their feeding vessel size, volume of the shunt, and drainage pattern [32,33]. Type I fistulae are small AVMs, the feeding artery and the draining vein are not dilated, and the shunt volume is low. Type II fistulae are medium sized AVMs fed by one or two dilated arteries, whereas type III fistulae harbor multiple massively dilated arterial feeders and a large shunt volume (Fig. 14). These latter fistulae are typically encountered in hereditary hemorrhagic telangiectasia (Figs. 15 and 16) [34,35].

Pathophysiologic mechanisms in spinal cord AVMs include venous congestion, and hemorrhage, space-occupying effects and a "steal phenomenon" also have been attributed to the pathogenesis [36,37]. If the AVM does not present initially with acute hemorrhage, symptomatology is unspecific. Patients may complain about hypo- or paraesthesia,

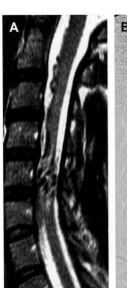
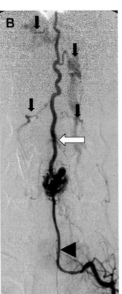
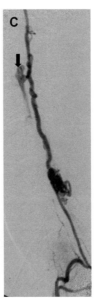

Fig. 11. Intramedullary spinal glomerular AVM at C5. (*A*) On T2-weighted MRI the intramedullary flow voids can be perceived. Slight cord edema is present in the vicinity. Ventral to the spinal cord, dilated vessels can be seen. (*B, C*) On angiography, an AVM supplied by the anterior spinal artery (*arrowhead*) arising from the left thyreocervical trunk can be perceived It drains exclusively cranially via an anterior spinal vein (white arrow), which subsequently drains into the epidural plexus at various levels (*black arrows*).

A   B   C

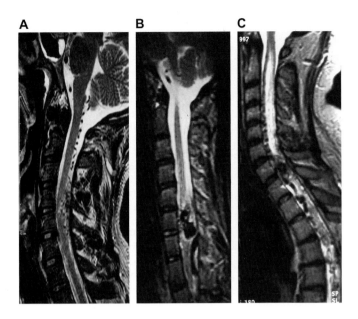

Fig. 12. Spectrum of imaging findings in three different patients with cervical intramedullary AVMs on T2-weighted images. (*A*) In the first patient, slightly dilated flow voids along the posterior aspect of the cord and at the level of C4 can be seen with moderate cord edema. (*B*) The second patient has an enlarged venous pouch and prominently enlarged draining veins (exclusively caudal) and no cord edema. (*C*) The third patient has a massive venous congestion of the cord and dilated veins along the ventral surface of the cord.

weakness, and diffuse back and muscle pain. Progressive sensorimotor symptoms can slowly develop or acutely worsen followed by improvements over time. Glomerular AVMs tend to be symptomatic in younger children and adolescents, whereas fistulous AVMs are symptomatic in young adults, the latter often presenting with a subarachnoid hemorrhage because of intradural location. Glomerular AVMs can become symptomatic by venous congestion alone [38], intraparenchymal hemorrhage, or a subarachnoid hemorrhage.

On MRI, the AVM type cannot be differentiated. The typical appearance of spinal cord AVMs is a conglomerate of dilated and peri- and intramedullarily located vessels that are demonstrated on T2-weighted sequences as flow voids. On T1-weighted sequences, depending on their flow velocity and direction, they are demonstrated as mixed

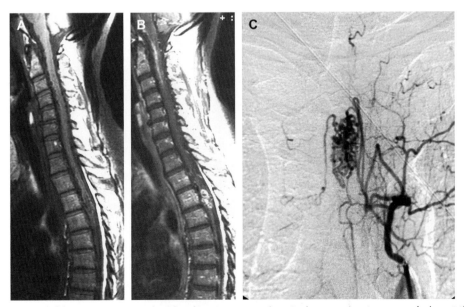

Fig. 13. A 47-yearold woman presented with subacute progressive ataxia, a sensory transverse lesion at the thoracic level, and sphincter disturbances. On pre- (*A*) and postcontrast (*B*) T1-weighted MRI, an enhancing lesion at the level of Th3 can be perceived. Pathologic flow voids indicate a spinal AVM, which was confirmed during selective spinal angiography (*C*).

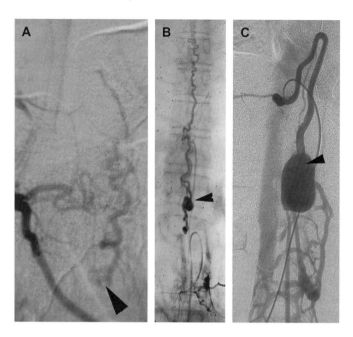

Fig. 14. Spectrum of angiographic imaging findings in perimedullary fistulae types 1 to 3. In type I (*A*), only a small feeding artery (in this case a dorsolateral artery) can be identified that directly (ie, without an intervening nidus) drains into perimedullary veins. This type can be differentiated from a dural AV fistula only by careful analysis of the point of fistulation (arrowhead) and the type of the feeding artery. In type II (*B*), a moderately enlarged radiculomedullary artery drains into a slightly enlarged venous pouch with subsequent cranial and caudal drainage. The shunting zone is demarcated by an arrowhead. In type III (*C*), a massively enlarged radiculomedullary artery drains into an enlarged venous pouch. This type of fistula always should raise suspicion of hereditary hemorrhagic telangiectasia.

hyper- and hypointense tubular structures. Contrast enhancement may vary. A venous congestive edema may be present as an intramedullary hyperintensity on T2-weighted images with concomitant swelling of the cord. The image might get even more complicated if intraparenchymal hemorrhages are present that might demonstrate varying signal intensities depending on the time elapsed between bleeding and imaging [39]. A subarachnoid hemorrhage might be present.

MRI should be able to identify the location of the AVM in relation to the cord and the dura. Especially in small perimedullary fistulous AVMs (type I), contrast media must be given to detect subtle venous dilatations [21,40,41]. Recently it was shown that fast MR angiography is capable of detecting the main arterial feeder of glomerular-type AVMs and perimedullary fistulous-type AVMs with a single large arterial feeder. Spinal cord AVMs with small or multiple feeders have not yet been investigated.

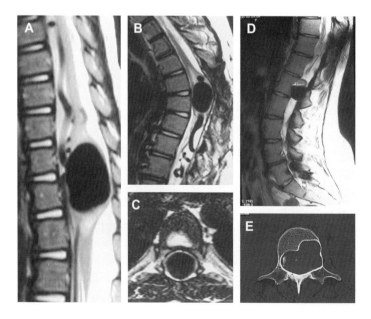

Fig. 15. Spectrum of imaging findings in type III spinal perimedullary AV fistulae (high shunting volume) in three patients (*A*, *B* + *C* and *D* + *E*, respectively). MRI can demonstrate the massively enlarged venous pouch and the dilated vessels in the vicinity. Cord edema is also present. On CT, bony erosions caused by the pulsating effect of the AVM can be perceived. All three patients harbored Rendu-Weber-Osler disease (hereditary hemorrhagic telangiectasia).

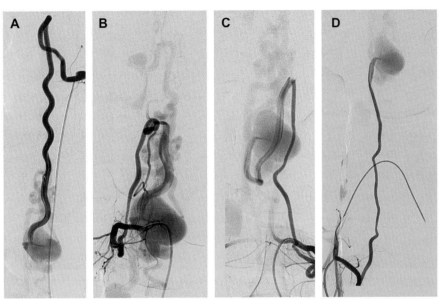

Fig. 16. Angiography in a spinal vascular malformation in a patient with hereditary hemorrhagic telangiectasia. The fistula can be classified as a type III perimedullary fistula with massively enlarged inflow and outflow tracts. A classic sign for hereditary hemorrhagic telangiectasia, a single hole AV fistula is present, with all different feeding arteries (*A–D*) draining at the same area into a massively enlarged venous pouch.

Selective spinal angiography remains necessary to define the exact type of the AVM and plan subsequent treatment.

The therapeutic approach of asymptomatic AVM is difficult because data concerning the spontaneous prognosis are not available; however, in symptomatic AVMs therapy ameliorates the prognosis of the patient. With the exception of the type I perimedullary fistula, the therapy of choice for all spinal cord AVMs is endovascular embolization with coils or glue after careful analysis of the selective spinal angiography [42].

In glomerular AVMs, glue or particles can be used to obliterate the nidus. Even a partial embolization seems to ameliorate the prognosis of the patient [16,43–45]. In type I perimedullary fistulae, the small caliber of the feeding artery may prohibit catheter placement close to the fistula; an operative treatment may then be favored. Types II and III fistulous AVMs, on the other hand, have dilated feeding vessels that enable superselective catheterization close to the fistula and subsequent closure (typically with concentrated glue or coils) [33,34].

Cavernomas

Spinal cord cavernomas (or cavernous malformations) are estimated to constitute 5% of all spinal vascular malformations [46,47]. Like their intracranial counterparts, cavernomas are discrete, lobulated, well-circumscribed, red to purple raspberry-like

lesions on gross pathology. Microscopically, these lesions are composed of dilated, thin-walled capillaries that have a simple endothelial lining with variably thin fibrous adventitia indistinguishable from the lining of a capillary telangiectasia [48]. Residua of previous hemorrhage, including scarring, collection of hemosiderin-laden macrophages, and calcification, may be present [49]. Typical clinical features of intramedullary cavernous malformations are sensory motor deficits, usually several hours after the onset of pain. The clinical course is variable, ranging from slowly progressive symptoms to acute quadriplegia. The acute setting is probably caused by new hemorrhage within or around the lesion. Repeated episodes of small bleedings or local pressure effect of the lesion itself on the surrounding spinal cord tissue by capillary proliferation, or vessel dilation may be responsible for slowly progressive symptoms.

Cavernomas appear as well-defined, circumscribed lesions of varying sizes that have a hypointense rim and an inhomogeneous, often hyperintense center on T2-weighted images. The hypointense rim is caused by magnetic susceptibility artifacts from hemosiderin deposits [50]. The complex reticulated core with its typical mulberry-like appearance represents hemorrhage in different stages of evolution (Figs. 17 and 18). CT might be of interest, because some cavernomas demonstrate extensive calcifications. Cavernomas are angiographically silent. In acutely hemorrhaged cavernomas, however, spinal

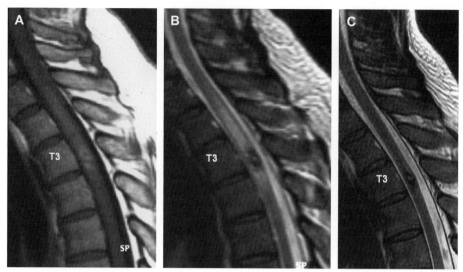

Fig. 17. Thoracic cavernoma of a 38-year-old man with acute onset of paraplegia. Sagittal T1- and T2-weighted MRI demonstrate an intramedullary lesion at the level of Th3 with a high central signal intensity on T1-weighted image (*A*). The lesion is hyperintense in the center surrounded by a hypointense zone and a perifocal hyperintense multi-segmental edema of the cord (T2-weighted image) (*B*). After 4 weeks, T2-weighted MRI (*C*) of the intramedullary lesion has a high central signal intensity (methemoglobin) and a hypointense rim (hemosiderin). Follow-up examinations identify the lesion as cavernoma with acute hemorrhage (histologically confirmed after surgery).

angiography should be performed to rule out that a small glomerular AVM, which might remain unnoticed on spinal MRI in the acute phase after a hemorrhage, was the culprit for the bleeding. Once the lesion becomes symptomatic, progressive myelopathy is the most common course [51].

Therapy is indicated. Surgical resection of cavernomas can be performed safely using meticulous microsurgical techniques. The localization of the cavernous malformation is mandatory to define the adequate operative strategy. Dissection is started directly over the lesion if the pathology approaches the surface of the cord. Deeply located lesions are either approached by a myelotomy performed over an area of bluish discoloration or by standard approaches (ie, through the dorsal root entry zone or by a midline myelotomy). Surgery is continued by gradual debulking of the mass. Dissection of the cavernous malformation is achieved by slight traction, coagulation, and gentle suction in the surrounding yellow plane of gliotic tissue preventing damage to the neighboring intact nervous tissue [51]. The lesion bed should be inspected carefully after resection for small residual portions.

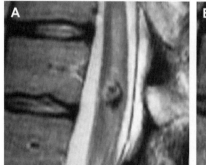
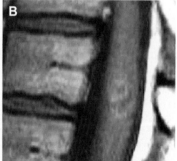
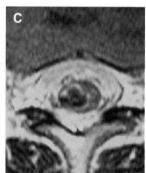

Fig. 18. Low thoracic cavernoma close to the conus medullaris. Although T2-weighted images (*A*, *C*) demonstrate the cavernoma better then the T1-weighted image (*B*), the size of the cavernoma is typically overestimated on T2 because of the hemosiderine present in the vicinity of the cavernoma. The mixed signal intensity on T1 and T2 represents blood degradation products at various stages.

Summary

The unspecific neurologic symptomatology and the variety of potentially detected vascular diseases make this clinical entity challenging for neurologists, neurosurgeons, and neuroradiologists. When spinal vascular diseases are suspected, MRI should constitute the first diagnostic modality to identify the lesion and rule out potential differential diagnoses (eg, acute cord compression, tumor, degenerative diseases of the spine, myelitis). Even with routine sequences, neuroradiologists should be able to detect intramedullary pathologies, such as intramedullary hemorrhages, cavernomas, edema or venous congestion, extramedullary intradural alterations (eg, dilated vessels or subarachnoidal hemorrhages), or potential extradural manifestations of spinal cord vascular malformations (eg, associated hemangiomas). MRA of the spinal cord constitutes a helpful adjunct to noninvasive diagnostics because it may demonstrate pathologic AV shunts and help to guide selective spinal arteriography.

When neurologic symptoms and MRI suggest a vascular malformation, spinal angiography is the next diagnostic step to define the type of vascular malformation, and decide about the appropriate therapy. Treatment in symptomatic patients offers an improvement in the prognosis but should be performed in specialized centers. Spinal cord cavernomas and type I perimedullary fistulae are surgical candidates. Dural AVMs can be operated on or treated by an endovascular approach. The former approach is simple, quick, and secure for obliterating fistulae, whereas the latter approach is technically demanding. In spinal AVMs the endovascular approach is the method of choice; in select cases a combined therapy might be sensible.

References

[1] Mull M, Thron A. Spinal infarcts. In: von Kummer R, Back T, editors. Magnetic resonance imaging in ischemic stroke. Berlin: Springer; 2006. p. 251–67.

[2] Thron A. Vascular anatomy of the spinal cord: neuroradiological investigations and clinical syndromes. Berlin: Springer; 1988.

[3] Lasjaunias PL, Berenstein A, terBrugge K. Surgical neuroangiography. In: Clinical vascular anatomy and variations, vol. 1. Berlin: Springer; 2001.

[4] Grunwald I, Thron A, Reith W. [Spinal angiography: vascular anatomy, technique and indications]. Radiologe 2001;41:961–7 [in German].

[5] Thron A, Otto J, Schroeder JM. Functional anatomy of the dural segment of spinal cord drainig veins: a histological and microangiographic study. In: du Boulay G, editor. Symposium neuroradiologicum. London: Springer-Verlag London Ltd.; 1990. p. 323.

[6] Gravereaux EC, Faries PL, Burks JA, et al. Risk of spinal cord ischemia after endograft repair of thoracic aortic aneurysms. J Vasc Surg 2001;34: 997–1003.

[7] Mikulis DJ, Ogilvy CS, McKee A, et al. Spinal cord infarction and fibrocartilagenous emboli. AJNR Am J Neuroradiol 1992;13:155–60.

[8] Rogopoulos A, Benchimol D, Paquis P, et al. Lumbar artery compression by the diaphragmatic crus: a new etiology for spinal cord ischemia. Ann Neurol 2000;48:261–4.

[9] Weidauer S, Nichtweiss M, Lanfermann H, et al. Spinal cord infarction: MR imaging and clinical features in 16 cases. Neuroradiology 2002;44: 851–7.

[10] Bammer R, Fazekas F, et al. Diffusion-weighted MR imaging of the spinal cord. AJNR Am J Neuroradiol 2000;21:587–91.

[11] Gass A, Back T, Behrens S, et al. MRI of spinal cord infarction. Neurology 2000;54:2195.

[12] Kueker W, Weller M, Klose U, et al. Diffusion weighted MRI of spinal cord infarction: high resolution and time course of diffusion abnormality. J Neurol 2004;251:818–24.

[13] Yuh WT, Marsh EE, Wang AK, et al. MR imaging of spinal cord and vertebral body infarction. AJNR Am J Neuroradiol 1992;13:145–54.

[14] Rodesch G, Hurth M, Alvarez H, et al. Classification of spinal cord arteriovenous shunts: proposal for a reappraisal. The Bicetre experience with 155 consecutive patients treated between 1981 and 1999. Neurosurgery 2002;51:374–9.

[15] Krings T, Mull M, Gilsbach JM, et al. Spinal vascular malformations. Eur Radiol 2005;15:267–78.

[16] Thron A, Caplan LR. Vascular malformations and interventional neuroradiology of the spinal cord. In: Brandt T, Caplan LR, Dichgans J, et al, editors. Neurological disorders course and treatment. Amsterdam: Academic Press; 2003. p. 517–28.

[17] Thron A. [Spinal dural arteriovenous fistulas]. Radiologe 2001;41:955–60 [in German].

[18] Hurst RW, Kenyon LC, Lavi E, et al. Spinal dural arteriovenous fistula: the pathology of venous hypertensive myelopathy. Neurology 1995;45: 1309–13.

[19] Criscuolo GR, Oldfield EH, Doppman JL. Reversible acute and subacute myelopathy in patients with dural arteriovenous fistulas: Foix-Alajouanine syndrome reconsidered. J Neurosurg 1989; 70:354–9.

[20] Bradac GB, Daniele D, Riva A, et al. Spinal dural arteriovenous fistulas: an underestimated cause of myelopathy. Eur Neurol 1994;34:87–94.

[21] Koenig E, Thron A, Schrader V, et al. Spinal arteriovenous malformations and fistulae: clinical, neuroradiological and neurophysiological findings. J Neurol 1989;236:260–6.

[22] Hurst RW, Grossman RI. Peripheral spinal cord hypointensity on T2-weighted MR images: a reliable imaging sign of venous hypertensive

myelopathy. AJNR Am J Neuroradiol 2000;21: 781–6.

[23] De Marco JK, Dillon WP, Halback VV, et al. Dural arteriovenous fistulas: evaluation with MR imaging. Radiology 1990;175:193–9.

[24] Huffmann BC, Gilsbach JM, Thron A. Spinal dural arteriovenous fistulas: a plea for neurosurgical treatment. Acta Neurochir (Wien) 1995; 135:44–51.

[25] Lee TT, Gromelski EB, Bowen BC, et al. Diagnostic and surgical management of spinal dural arteriovenous fistulas. Neurosurgery 1998;43: 242–6; [discussion: 246–7].

[26] Niimi Y, Berenstein A, Setton A, et al. Embolization of spinal dural arteriovenous fistulae: results and follow-up. Neurosurgery 1997;40:675–82; [discussion: 682–3].

[27] Rodesch G, Hurth M, Alvarez H, et al. Spinal cord intradural arteriovenous fistulae: anatomic, clinical, and therapeutic considerations in a series of 32 consecutive patients seen between 1981 and 2000 with emphasis on endovascular therapy. Neurosurgery 2005;57:973–83.

[28] Van Dijk JM, TerBrugge KG, Willinsky RA, et al. Multidisciplinary management of spinal dural arteriovenous fistulas: clinical presentation and long-term follow-up in 49 patients. Stroke 2002;33:1578–83.

[29] Behrens S, Thron A. Long-term follow-up and outcome in patients treated for spinal dural arteriovenous fistula. J Neurol 1999;246:181–5.

[30] Rosenblum B, Oldfield EH, Doppman JL, et al. Spinal arteriovenous malformations: a comparison of dural arteriovenous fistulas and intradural AVMs in 81 patients. J Neurosurg 1987;67: 795–802.

[31] Heros RC, Debrun GM, Ojemann RG, et al. Direct spinal arteriovenous fistula: a new type of spinal AVM [case report]. J Neurosurg 1986; 64:134–9.

[32] Gueguen B, Merland JJ, Riche MC, et al. Vascular malformations of the spinal cord: intrathecal perimedullary arteriovenous fistulas fed by medullary arteries. Neurology 1987;37:969–79.

[33] Mourier KL, Gobin YP, George B, et al. Intradural perimedullary arteriovenous fistulae: results of surgical and endovascular treatment in a series of 35 cases. Neurosurgery 1993;32:885–91; [discussion: 891].

[34] Krings T, Chng SM, Ozanne A, et al. Hereditary hemorrhagic telangiectasia in children: endovascular treatment of neurovascular malformations. Results in 31 patients. Neuroradiology 2005;47: 946–54.

[35] Krings T, Ozanne A, Chng SM, et al. Neurovascular phenotypes in hereditary haemorrhagic telangiectasia patients according to age: review of 50 consecutive patients aged 1 day-60 years. Neuroradiology 2005;47:711–20.

[36] Aminoff MJ, Logue V. Clinical features of spinal vascular malformations. Brain 1974;97:197–210.

[37] Aminoff MJ, Logue V. The prognosis of patients with spinal vascular malformations. Brain 1974; 97:211–8.

[38] Kataoka H, Miyamoto S, Nagata I, et al. Venous congestion is a major cause of neurological deterioration in spinal arteriovenous malformations. Neurosurgery 2001;48:1224–9; [discussion: 1229–30].

[39] Gomori JM, Grossman RI, Yu-Ip C, et al. NMR relaxation times of blood: dependence on field strength, oxidation state, and cell integrity. J Comput Assist Tomogr 1987;11:684–90.

[40] Doppman JL, Di Chiro G, Dwyer AJ, et al. Magnetic resonance imaging of spinal arteriovenous malformations. J Neurosurg 1987;66:830–4.

[41] Thron A, Mull M, Reith W. [Spinal arteriovenous malformations]. Radiologe 2001;41:949–54 [in German].

[42] Biondi A, Merland JJ, Reizine D, et al. Embolization with particles in thoracic intramedullary arteriovenous malformations: long-term angiographic and clinical results. Radiology 1990; 177:651–8.

[43] Doppman JL, Di Chiro G, Ommaya A. Obliteration of spinal-cord arteriovenous malformation by percutaneous embolisation. Lancet 1968;1:477.

[44] Djindjian R, Cophignon J, Rey A, et al. Superselective arteriographic embolization by the femoral route in neuroradiology: study of 50 cases. II. Embolization in vertebromedullary pathology. Neuroradiology 1973;6:132–42.

[45] Rodesch G, Hurth M, Alvarez H, et al. Embolization of spinal cord arteriovenous shunts: morphological and clinical follow-up and results. Review of 69 consecutive cases. Neurosurgery 2003;53:40–9.

[46] Spetzger U, Gilsbach JM, Bertalanffy H. Cavernous angiomas of the spinal cord: clinical presentation, surgical strategy, and postoperative results. Acta Neurochir (Wien) 1995;134:200–6.

[47] Zevgaridis D, Medele RJ, Hamburger C, et al. Cavernous haemangiomas of the spinal cord: a review of 117 cases. Acta Neurochir (Wien) 1999;141:237–45.

[48] Rigamonti D, Johnson PC, Spetzler RF, et al. Cavernous malformations and capillary telangiectasia: a spectrum within a single pathological entity. Neurosurgery 1991;28:60–4.

[49] Russell DS, Rubinstein LJ. Pathology of tumours of the nervous system. Baltimore (MD): Williams & Wilkins; 1989.

[50] Weinzierl MR, Krings T, Korinth MC, et al. MRI and intraoperative findings in cavernous haemangiomas of the spinal cord. Neuroradiology 2004;46:65–71.

[51] Anson JA, Spetzler RF. Surgical resection of intramedullary spinal cord cavernous malformations. J Neurosurg 1993;78:446–51.

NEUROIMAGING
CLINICS
OF NORTH AMERICA

Neuroimag Clin N Am 17 (2007) 73–85

Spinal Trauma

Pia C. Sundgren, MD, PhD[a],*, Marcel Philipp, MD[b],
Pavel V. Maly, MD, PhD[c]

- Imaging modalities
  Plain film radiography
  CT
  MR imaging
- Criteria for imaging and choice of imaging modality
- Types of injuries
  Cervical spine injuries
  Thoracic and lumbar spine injuries
- Trauma to the spinal cord and spinal content

- *Spinal cord injuries*
  Traumatic disc herniation
  Ligamentous injury
- Trauma to the pediatric spine
- Late posttraumatic changes in the spinal cord
- Summary
- Acknowledgments
- References

Injuries to the spinal column and the spinal cord are a major cause of disability, affecting predominantly young, healthy individuals. Approximately 30,000 spinal injuries occur in the United States every year. Up to 60% of the injuries affect young, healthy males between 15 and 35 years of age. Therefore, the socioeconomic consequences are important, and the costs of lifetime care and rehabilitation are extremely high, often more than $1,000,000 per individual [1].

Most spinal trauma involves cervical spine injuries, with more than 10,000 cervical fractures and more than 4000 thoracolumbar fractures diagnosed per year. The main cause for spinal injuries is blunt trauma, most commonly caused by motor vehicle accidents (48%), followed by falls (21%) and sport injuries (14.6%). Assault and penetrating trauma account for approximately 10% to 20% of cases. Almost one half of spinal injuries result in

neurologic deficits, which are often severe and sometimes fatal [2]. Survival is inversely related to the patient's age, and the mortality rate during initial hospitalization is reported to be almost 10% [3].

Injury to the spinal cord occurs in 10% to 14% of spinal fractures and dislocations [4]. Injuries of the cervical spine are by far the most common cause of neurologic deficits, which occur in almost 40% of the cases [5]. Most (85%) injuries to the spinal cord occur at the time of trauma, and 5% to 10% are present in the immediate postinjury period [6].

Imaging modalities

Plain film radiography

In cases where multislice CT (MSCT) is not available, plain film radiographs remain the initial imaging modality. To clear the cervical spine,

[a] Department of Radiology, University of Michigan Health Systems, 1500 East Medical Center Drive, Ann Arbor, MI 48104, USA
[b] Department of Radiology, Medical University Vienna, Waehringer Guertel 18-20, A-1090 Vienna, Austria
[c] Department of Radiology, University Hospital MAS, University of Lund, Malmoe, Sweden
* Corresponding author.
E-mail address: sundgren@umich.edu (P.C. Sundgren).

a minimum of three sets of views must be obtained: a lateral, an anteroposterior, and an open-mouth, odontoid view. Often, additional views, such as oblique views or the swimmer's view, are performed in an attempt to clear the cervicothoracic junction. Flexion and extension views are contraindicated in the acute setting. They usually do not add any additional information [7], and, in the acute setting, cases of unstable ligamentous injury may be masked by neck pain and muscle spasm, which limit the range of motion on extension-flexion views [8]. The potential benefit of flexion and extension views is in the subacute setting 2 to 4 weeks after the trauma, to rule out delayed cervical instability [9].

The presence of neurologic deficits, back pain, and a Glasgow Coma Score of eight or less gives an overall sensitivity of almost 100% for the clinical evaluation of spinal trauma in the setting of blunt trauma [10,11]. Overall, the sensitivity of plain films in diagnosing spinal injuries, especially injuries in the cervical spine, varies, ranging from 39% to 94%, with variable specificity [11–17]. Several studies have proved that if only plain radiographs are used, 23% to 57% of all fractures of the cervical spine are missed [14,18,19]. Delays in the diagnosis of clinically significant cervical spine injuries have been reported in approximately 5% to 23% of patients in various series, most of which used plain films as the initial screening modality.

CT

Today, MSCT (or single-slice helical CT) is the initial method of choice when evaluating the cervical spine for bone injuries after blunt trauma [14,20–25]. CT not only detects fractures with higher sensitivity than plain films, but can detect soft tissue abnormalities, such as disc herniation and paravertebral soft tissue and intraspinal hematoma. MSCT allows whole-spine examination in a very short time, and fast reformatting of images in multiple planes allows for a better and more exact diagnosis of bone and soft tissue abnormalities. With the introduction of these new CT imaging techniques, most trauma centers have set up dedicated, acute, multitrauma protocols that include CT of the brain, cervical spine, thorax, and abdomen, with subsequent reformatting of images of the thoracic and lumbar spine. In addition, several institutions have completely replaced plain films with MSCT in blunt spinal trauma patients, especially for the cervical spine, including two- and three-dimensional reformatting. The use of axial CT only is obsolete because of its limitations in demonstrating subluxations, increased intervertebral distances, angulations, or horizontal fractures. One study demonstrated that axial CT only detected 54% of

dislocations and subluxations in trauma patients [26].

Typically, (spiral) MSCT in high-resolution mode with 1.25- to 2-mm–thin slices in the C1-C2 region, 2- to 3-mm–thin slices in the rest of the cervical spine and 3- to 4-mm–thin slices in the thoracic and lumbar spine are chosen for axial presentation. Sagittal and coronal reformatted images of the entire spine are produced from contiguous, submillimeter (0.3–0.75 mm) axial images, or, on the older scanners, from thicker slices that have been reconstructed with overlapping (eg, at 1.5 mm). In addition to reconstructions with bone algorithm, reconstructing images with soft tissue algorithm has been proposed to facilitate the evaluation of, for example, intra-and extraspinal hemorrhage or disc herniation.

MR imaging

MR imaging is the imaging modality of choice for assessing soft tissue injuries, spinal cord injury, intervertebral discs and ligaments, and vascular injuries [27–29]. MR imaging is the only method that can differentiate spinal cord hemorrhage from edema, which might be of prognostic significance and possibly may change the treatment (Fig. 1). MR imaging is the examination of choice for excluding instability, proving or excluding cord or disc injury in patients who have focal neurologic signs, and for those who need preoperative spinal canal clearance before surgery. Compromise of the spinal canal and neural foramina, and cord compression in the presence or absence of an acute fracture, also can be evaluated sufficiently with MR imaging. MR imaging allows for better differentiation between acute and chronic compression fractures and bone marrow abnormalities. In addition, posttraumatic sequelae, such as syrinx formation, myelomalacia, and cord atrophy or tethering, typically are examined and evaluated with MR imaging. Performing MR imaging involves some safety issues, especially in assaulted patients who have penetrating injuries. The possibility for bullet or other metallic fragments close to the spinal canal to move and cause cord injury has to be considered [30,31]. However, the results of some small series have shown no adverse effects in patients who have bullets within, or in close proximity to, the spinal canal [32]. Because many patients who have suspected spinal injury are severely and critically ill, issues with halos or ventilators, the need for monitoring during scanning, and the presence of other extensive serious injuries to the brain, chest, or abdomen have to be considered; MR imaging–compatible devices have to be used when these patients are brought to the MR imaging unit. Today, these safety issues can be handled in most cases.

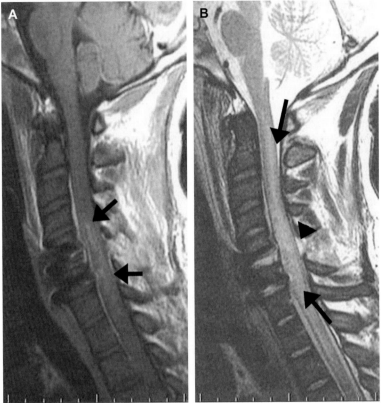

Fig. 1. Sagittal T1-weighted and T2-weighted MR images in a young man, status postsurgical anterior fusion after C5-C6 fracture after wrestling accident. Sagittal T1-weighted image (*A*) shows increased signal in the cervical cord (*arrows*), consistent with hemorrhage, and the T2-weighted image (*B*) demonstrates increased T2 signal in the cervical cord from C2 to C7 caused by edema (*arrows*); rupture of the interspinous ligament is also evident (*arrowhead*).

However, most centers use MR imaging as an additional modality, and have a dedicated spine trauma MR imaging protocol, which includes several of the following sequences:

- Sagittal T2 short-T1 inversion recovery (STIR), T2-weighted, and T1-weighted images, pre- and postcontrast
- Axial T1-weighted images, pre- and postcontrast
- Axial T2-weighted, fat-saturated images for ligamentous and soft tissue injuries
- T2* gradient echo images to evaluate for small hemorrhage or blood products in the spinal cord

Criteria for imaging and choice of imaging modality

One of the critical decisions in the emergency clinical setting is determining which patients require imaging of the spine. Different studies have tried to separate low-risk from high-risk patients

[12,33,34]. The National Emergency X-Radiology Utilization Study (NEXUS) established five criteria to classify the patients having a low probability of injury [33]. These criteria included no midline cervical tenderness, no focal neurologic deficit, normal alertness, no intoxication, and the absence of a painful distracting injury. The negative predictive value of this tool was 99.8% [10], but with a low specificity value of only 12%. Other retrospective studies have found the NEXUS low-risk criteria to be less sensitive (92.7%) but to have a higher specificity, 37.8% [34]. Another, perhaps more sensitive or more accurate, method is the Canadian C-spine rule [11,34]. The Canadian C-spine rule divides patients into high-risk versus low-risk patients, based on the presence of high-risk factors that mandates radiography, or the presence of any low-risk factor that allows the safe assessment of a range of motion. The high-risk factors are 65 or more years of age, dangerous mechanism, or paresthesias in extremities. The low-risk factors include simple rear-end motor vehicle collision, a sitting position in the emergency department, whether the patient has been ambulatory at any time since the trauma, the delayed onset of neck pain, or the absence of mid-line cervical spine tenderness. In addition, patients in a recent study were evaluated as to whether they were able to rotate their necks 45° to the left and right, by cross-validation, this rule had a 100% sensitivity and a 42.5% specificity for identifying clinically important cervical spine fractures [11].

The choice of modality depends on several factors, such as the availability of the different imaging modalities, the patient's clinical and neurologic condition, the type of trauma (blunt, single, or multitrauma), other associated injuries to the brain, thorax, or abdomen, complaints of pain or limited neck or spine motion, the presence of permanent or transient neurologic deficits, and, finally, the reason for the examination (high clinical suspicion of spinal injury versus just a question of excluding injury for legal reasons in a patient with very low suspicion). A special group of patients is composed of those who need spinal cord and spinal canal clearance before surgery, in which case MR imaging is the method of choice.

Negative plain films do not exclude fractures in the craniocervical junction (ie, C1 or C2) or in the cervicothoracic junction, or soft tissue injury in the craniocervical junction, or, in these cases, the liberal use of CT or MR imaging is recommended. MR imaging is recommended also if the patient complains of pain in the setting of negative plain films. MR imaging should be performed also if the patient has symptoms that cannot be explained by the plain film or CT radiologic findings, to evaluate for intraspinal soft tissue injuries, traumatic disc herniations, or cord abnormalities.

Types of injuries

The spine is divided into three osteoligamentous columns: anterior, middle, and posterior. The anterior column includes the anterior longitudinal ligament and the anterior two thirds of the vertebral body and disc, including annulus fibrosus. The components of the middle column are the posterior third of the vertebral body and disc, including annulus fibrosus, and the posterior longitudinal ligament. The posterior column is composed of the pedicles, articular processes, facet capsules, laminae, ligamenta flava, spinous processes, and interspinous ligaments. Depending on the mechanism of injury, several different types of traumatic injuries to the cervical, and the thoracic and lumbar spine, may occur, which may result in stable or unstable spine injuries. The two- or three-column concept [35–38] was applied initially only to the lower thoracic and lumbar spine but can, with some

modifications, be applied also to the cervical spine. Basically, the three-column concept states that fractures affecting more than two of the three columns, or only the middle column, are unstable, and the blunt trauma can be classified therefore by the anatomic location and the biomechanics of the injury.

Several studies have analyzed a more general pattern of spinal injury, and the correlation between type of trauma and type of fracture in the overall population, in the elderly, and in children [39–41]. Burst fractures are the most common spine injuries after a fall, with 50% located in the thoracolumbar junction, followed by compression fractures [41]. Cervical spine injuries are twice as common in patients older than 70, compared with the nongeriatric population, and odontoid fractures are the most frequent fracture, accounting for 20% of all fractures. In children younger than nine, the most commonly injured level is the higher cervical spine, whereas older children more commonly have injuries to the lower cervical spine [40,42].

Cervical spine injuries

Cervical spine injury can be divided simplistically into three major groups, based on the biomechanics behind the injury: hyperflexion injuries, hyperextension injuries, and vertical compression injuries.

Hyperflexion injuries include anterior subluxation, bilateral interfacetal dislocation, simple wedge fracture, clay-shoveller's fracture (fracture of the spinous process), teardrop fracture, and odontoid (dens) fracture (Figs. 2–4). The bilateral interfacet dislocation and the teardrop fracture are considered unstable. The odontoid fracture can be considered stable or unstable, depending on the fracture type. The remaining injuries are considered stable. The mechanism behind the flexion injury of the cervical and thoracolumbar spine results in forward rotation or translation of the vertebral body and, secondarily, compression in the anterior column with distraction in the posterior column. The injury is caused by forces that cause hyperflexion of the spine in the neutral position, or by a direct trauma to the flexed head and neck. This type of mechanism results in disruption of the posterior and interlaminar ligaments, the facet capsules, and the posterior part of the annulus fibrosus. Hyperflexion fractures often are associated with traumatic disc herniation.

Hyperextension injuries are less frequent than hyperflexion injuries, and usually are the result of an anterior impact to the face, forehead, or mandible, or sudden deceleration as the underlying mechanism. Hyperextension trauma results in the following types of injuries: dislocation, avulsion fracture or fracture of the posterior arch of C1, teardrop fracture of C2, laminar fracture, and the so-called Hangman's fracture. Most of these injuries, with the exception of Hangman's fracture, are considered stable. The Hangman's fracture involves C2 and can be divided into three types, depending on the location of the fracture [43]. Because at least two columns are disrupted in the Hangman's fracture, this fracture is considered unstable. Hyperextension injuries often are associated with central cord syndrome, in the form of cord edema or diffuse prevertebral soft tissue swelling.

Finally, the Jefferson fracture involves the atlas and is considered unstable. The Jefferson fracture and the burst fracture are caused by vertical compression (Fig. 5). Burst fractures are either stable or unstable, and may cause spinal cord injuries in up to 50% of cases because of encroachment on the spinal canal (Fig. 6). Cusick and Yoganandan [44] presented a more detailed classification of injury and the biomechanisms of injury. The diagnosis of whiplash injury or whiplash-associated disorder is determined by clinical history, the mechanism of injury, and the symptoms and neurologic findings at examination. Whiplash injury is increasingly common and frequently is caused by rear-end motor vehicle accidents, with hyperextension and hyperflexion of the neck. Symptoms include neck pain, neck stiffness, paresthesias, upper extremity pain, jaw pain, and headache. Most imaging

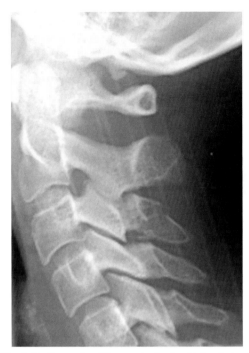

Fig. 2. Radiograph of the cervical spine (lateral view), demonstrating an isolated C3 spinous process fracture. The isolated spinous process fracture is considered a stable fracture. These fractures can be hard to see on axial CT images because the imaging plane is the same as the plane of the fracture line.

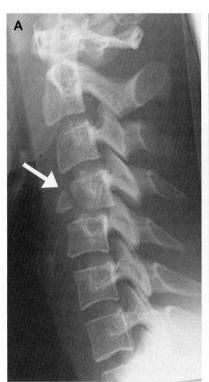

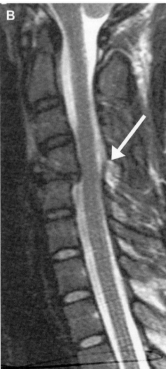

Fig. 3. Radiograph of cervical spine (lateral) demonstrates flexion teardrop fracture (*arrow*) in C4 vertebral body with mild posterior displacement of the C4 vertebral body in comparison to C5 (*A*). Sagittal T2-weighted MR imaging demonstrates mild flattening of the anterior aspect of the cervical cord and rupture of the posterior ligament (*arrow*), but no T2 signal hyperintensity in the cord to suggest cord injury (*B*).

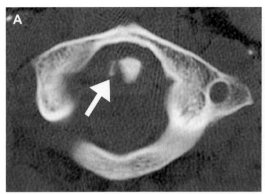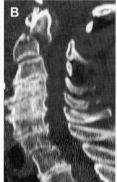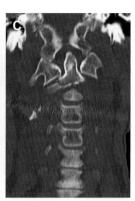

Fig. 4. The odontoid fractures can be divided into three types, depending on the injury: avulsion of the tip of the dens (type 1) (*arrow*) (*A*), fracture through the base of the dens (type II) (*B*), and fracture through the corpus (type III) (*C*).

techniques in patients who have suspected whiplash injury are inconclusive [45]. The role of imaging in the work-up of patients who have whiplash injury remains controversial and possibly not cost-effective, at least in the acute stage [46–48]. Most patients report recovery, with a resolution of symptoms. Some whiplash patients do develop chronic neck pain [1,49,50] and in these patients who have persistent symptoms, imaging might play a role. A recent study found eight disc herniations in 24 patients who had symptoms for more than 6 weeks after trauma [51].

Thoracic and lumbar spine injuries

The fractures in the lower thoracic and lumbar spine are often complex and are caused by a combination of mechanisms. The most common fracture is the simple compression or wedge fracture (50% of all fractures), which is stable. The remaining types of fractures are considered unstable. The wedge fracture is a compression of the anterior vertebral body, more prominent in the superior end plate, and is considered stable if the angulation is less than 40°. Several variants of flexion injuries with distraction in the thoracic and lumbar spine are recognized; the most common is the so-called "seat beat injury," which can be divided into three subtypes, depending on injury [52]. Type I (Chance fracture) involves the posterior bony elements, type II (Smith fracture) involves the posterior ligaments, and, in type III, the annulus fibrosus is ruptured, allowing for subluxation [52].

Burst fractures most commonly occur in the thoracolumbar region, accounting for 64% to 81% of all thoracolumbar fractures, and are associated with a high incidence of injuries to the spinal cord, conus medullaris, cauda equina, and nerve roots [53]. Burst fractures can be divided into five subtypes: fractures of both superior and inferior end plates; fracture of the superior end plate; fracture

of the inferior end plate; burst rotation; and lateral flexion fractures [54]. Burst fractures are recognized by a combination of wedge compression of the anterior column and fractures of the posterior cortex (which is part of the middle column) with retropulsion of fracture fragments into the spinal canal (Fig. 7). On plain films, burst fractures can be misdiagnosed as mere compression fractures [55]. Because of that, an unstable burst fracture that involves the anterior and middle columns can be treated erroneously as a stable compression or as a mild wedge fracture that involves only the anterior column.

Trauma to the spinal cord and spinal content

Spinal cord injuries

The United States Major Trauma Outcome Study estimated the incidence of acute spinal cord injury to

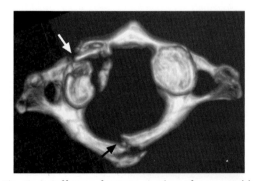

Fig. 5. A Jefferson fracture consists of an unstable fracture of the C1 ring caused by an axial loading injury to the head with compression force to C1 (typically from diving). Three-dimensional reformatted CT images demonstrate unilateral fractures of the anterior (*white arrow*) and posterior (*black arrow*) arches of C1.

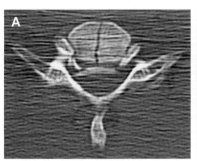
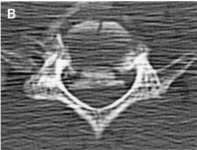
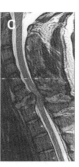

Fig. 6. Axial CT (*A* and *B*) demonstrates fracture through the C7 vertebral body and displacement of fracture fragment posteriorly with narrowing of the spinal canal in 21-year-old man with a vertical compression fracture of C7 vertebral body after a diving accident. Sagittal T2-weighted MR imaging (*C*) shows the compressed C7 vertebral body and increased T2 signal in the cervical cord caused by cord injury.

be 2.6% of blunt trauma patients [56]. The costs for treating an individual with traumatic spinal cord injury are estimated to be between $500,000 and $2 million (US dollars), depending on factors such as the extent and location of injury. The total direct costs of caring for individuals with spinal cord injury exceed $7 billion per year in the United States [57].

The pathophysiology to spinal cord injuries has nicely been described previously [57] and can be summarized as a primary injury caused by direct compression or neural elements by bony fracture fragments, disc material and ligamentous injuries, and from associated epidural hematoma or disruption or transection of the cord due to penetrating trauma (gun bullets or weapons). Damage occurs to the blood vessels, axons are disrupted, and microhemorrhages occur within minutes in the central gray matter and spread out within the next hours. The spinal cord swells within minutes after the injury and, when the cord swelling exceeds the venous pressure, secondary ischemia occurs. The ischemia and release of toxic chemicals from disrupted neural membranes trigger a second injury that results in a spinal shock and kills neighboring cells [57]. Our understanding of what happens secondarily is limited, but recent data suggest that cell death occurs days to weeks after the injury, with apoptosis of the oligodendrocytes not only at the site of injury but also several levels away from the injury site [58].

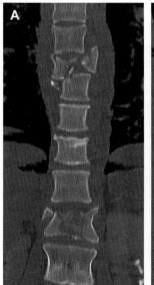
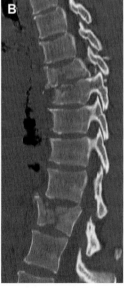
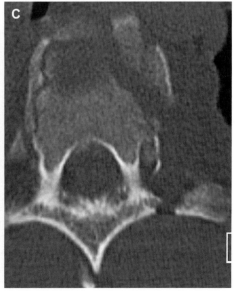

Fig. 7. A 41-year-old woman, status post-motor vehicle accident, admitted to the emergency room with paraplegia. Coronal (*A*) and sagittal (*B*) images demonstrate multiple burst fractures in the thoracic spine, with additional anterior wedge fracture and superior end plate fracture. Dorsal displacement of fracture fragments is present. Axial image demonstrates the burst vertebral body at the end plate level.

The assessment of the spinal cord injury patient includes evaluation of mental status, cranial nerves, motor and sensory function, autonomic systems co-ordination, and gait. Nearly all spinal cord injuries damage upper and lower motor neurons. The severity of the injury can be defined by the American Spinal Injury Association's five-level impairment scale: grade A, no sensory or motor function preserved in the sacral segments S4-S5 (complete); grade B, sensory function preserved, but no motor function below the neurologic level and extending through the sacral segments S4-S5 (incomplete); grades C and D, both considered incomplete, with motor function preserved below the neurologic level, with most key muscles having a grade of less than three (grade C) or greater than three (grade D); and grade E, normal motor and sensory function. Spinal-cord injury also has other international standards of neurologic and functional classifications [59,60].

The symptoms of complete spinal cord transaction depend on the level of injury. A high cervical injury results in respiratory insufficiency, quadriplegia with upper and lower extremity areflexia, loss of sphincter tone, and anesthesia caused by neurogenic shock. If the injury is located in the lower cervical spine, the patient's respiratory function is preserved. Higher thoracic lesions cause paraplegia or quadriparesis. Lower thoracic and lumbar/sacral injuries present with urinary and bowel retention. The cause for transection is often fracture with dislocation of the spinal vertebral bodies, but penetrating trauma with weapons and gun bullets also can result in transection of the spinal cord (Fig. 8).

Incomplete spinal cord injuries are further categorized clinically into anterior cord syndrome, Brown-Sequard syndrome, central cord syndrome, conus medullaris syndrome, cauda equina syndrome, and spinal cord contusions. Anterior cord syndrome is seen typically with anterior spinal artery infarction, and results in variable loss of motor function, and pain and temperature, with relative sparing of proprioception below the level of the lesion. Anterior cord syndrome has the worst prognosis of all cord syndromes, with only 10-% to 15% of patients demonstrating functional recovery. The prognosis is good if recovery is evident and progressive during the first 24 hours after injury.

Brown-Sequard syndrome is common after trauma and is more or less the same as hemicordectomy, with ipsilateral paralysis and position sense below the level of injury, hyperreflexia and extensor toe sign occurring at the level of injury, and loss of pain and temperature on contralateral side a few segments below the level of the lesion.

Hyperextension injury might result in a hemorrhage in the central part of the spinal cord and destruction of the axons in the lateral columns at the level of injury to the spinal cord, with relative sparring of the gray matter, which can cause acute traumatic central cord syndrome, characterized by disproportionately greater motor impairment in the upper extremities, compared with lower bladder dysfunction and a variable degree of sensory loss below the level of injury, and with considerable recovery. Central cord syndrome often occurs in the elderly, with cervical spondylosis after hyperextension injury caused by buckled ligamenta flava or osteophytes impinging on the posterior cord, but can occur with any type of injury mechanism and in any age group.

The cauda equina and conus medullaris syndromes present with polyradiculopathy, with sensory changes, asymmetric, lower motor neuron–type leg weakness, and sphincter disturbances; lesions in the conus medullaris also cause early disturbance of the bowel and bladder function.

Recovery from spinal cord injury, if it occurs, happens within the first 6 months; patients commonly regain one level of motor function, with retention of sacral sensation and age being two significant prognostic factors [58,61,62].

Traumatic disc herniation

Traumatic disc herniation should be considered when the disc has a high signal on T2-weighted images or when severe traumatic vertebral body fractures or ligamentous injury is present [63]. Traumatic disc herniation commonly is caused by distraction and shearing in sudden extension, but can also occur in flexion injuries (Fig. 9). Cervical disc herniations are seen in 54% to 80% of patients who have facet dislocation [64].

The sensitivity for detecting traumatic disc herniations with MR imaging is high, but the specificity is low [64].

Ligamentous injury

The major ligaments in the spine are the anterior and posterior longitudinal ligaments, the ligamenta flava, the interspinous ligament, and the ligamentum nuchae. In the craniocervical junction, three additional stabilizing ligaments are present: the tectorial membrane, the transverse ligament, and the alar ligaments. Ligamentous injury can be suspected on plain films or CT in patients who have malalignment of vertebral bodies, or dislocation or subluxation of vertebral bodies and facets after blunt trauma [65]. Despite the introduction of helical MSCT, which is the method of choice for screening and detecting cervical spine bone injuries, MR imaging is the best imaging method for evaluating the spinal content and allows for direct visualization of the ligamentous structures and their injuries [65,66]. However, the sensitivity of MR imaging in

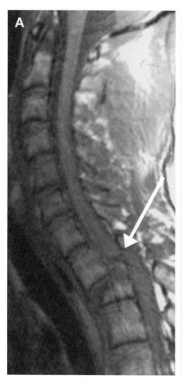
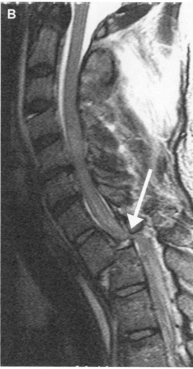

Fig. 8. A 35-year-old female paraplegic after a motor vehicle accident with flexion extension injury, posterior lamina fractures, and facet fractures and dislocation of T1-T2 vertebral bodies, resulting in cord transection. Sagittal T1-weighted (*A*) and T2-weighted (*B*) images demonstrate the transected cord (*arrows*) at the level of injury, and signal abnormalities in the cervical and upper thoracic cord.

detecting ligamentous injuries is relatively low, around 55% to 65% [65,67]. In a recent study comparing helical CT with MR imaging, 21 of 85 patients (25%) had ligamentous injury identified on MR imaging. Of these 21 patients, 14 patients (66.6%) had ligamentous injuries only identified on MR imaging [65].

Ligamentous injury has to be suspected when there is a gap between parts of the vertebrae or when there is increased signal in the ligament or adjacent structures on T2-weighted and STIR images. In a recent study, ligamentous injury was present in 11 of 17 patients who had prevertebral space signal abnormalities with no fracture or dislocation; no instability was seen in those who had no prevertebral signal abnormalities [68]. Ligamentous injury without underlying fracture in the cervical spine is rare [65,69]. Often, disruption of the anterior longitudinal ligament is seen in hyperextension injuries, with associated injury to the prevertebral muscles and intervertebral discs, and may have a poor clinical outcome if not treated surgically to prevent instability. It can be seen as an interruption of the normal linear band of hypointense signal of the ligament on T1-weighted images. Disruption of the posterior ligamentous complex is caused by distraction and flexion forces and is manifested by increased distance between interspinous processes during flexion (Fig. 10).

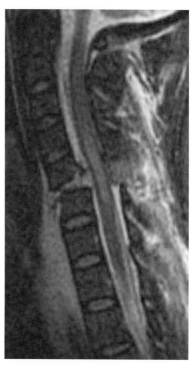

Fig. 9. Sagittal T2-weighted MR imaging of the cervical spine in a 45-year-old female pedestrian hit by a car demonstrates ventral subluxation of C5 on C6 vertebral body, with posterior disc herniation and cord compression and edema in the cervical cord, extending from mid-C4 to mid-C6 vertebral body levels.

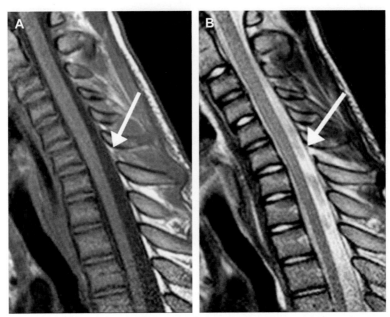

Fig. 10. Sagittal T1-weighted (*A*) and T2-weighted (*B*) MR imaging in a 15-year-old boy after high-speed rollover motor vehicle crash demonstrates increased distances between spinous processes, rupture of the interspinous ligament (*arrows*), and posterior soft tissue injury at the C6-C7 level. (*Courtesy of* Dr. S. Gujar, Department of Radiology, University of Michigan, Ann Arbor, MI.)

Trauma to the pediatric spine

Injuries to the spine and spinal cord are relatively infrequent in the pediatric population [70–73], and about 40% to 60% of them occur in the cervical spine. Upper cervical spine fractures are more frequent in children under the age of nine, whereas lower cervical spine injuries are more frequent in older children. The most common cause of spine injuries varies with the age of the patient. In infants and children up to three years old, motor vehicle accidents, obstetric complications, falls, and child abuse are the most common causes for spine injury. In children 3 to 10 years of age, falls and bicycle and auto-pedestrian accidents account for most injuries [74,75]. In children 10 years and older, sports, diving accidents, and motor vehicle accidents account for most injuries [76,77]. Injuries caused by violence and penetrating injuries are far less common than in adults.

Spinal cord injury in children often occurs without evidence of fracture or dislocation [78] because of the inherent elasticity of the vertebral column of infants and young children, which makes the cord vulnerable to injury. Spinal cord injury without radiographic abnormality often has a poor long-term prognosis. Pediatric cervical injuries more often involve the ligaments; children are also more prone to spinal cord injuries, often without plain film abnormalities, compared with adults.

Late posttraumatic changes in the spinal cord

In patients who have severe spinal trauma with cord injuries, development of spinal cord atrophy and myelomalacia are the most common findings (62% and 54%, respectively), followed by syrinx (22%), spinal cord cysts (9%), and transection of the cord (7%) [79]. In addition, tethering or adhesions of the cord can be seen after traumatic spinal injury [80].

Summary

Injuries to the spine and its contents affect predominately young, healthy individuals and are a major cause of disability, with significant socioeconomic consequences. Already, in the initial evaluation of patients who have blunt trauma, MSCT with two-dimensional (and three-dimensional) reformatting is the method of choice. The liberal use of MR imaging is recommended to assess for injuries to soft tissue, the spine and its contents, intervertebral discs, and ligaments.

Acknowledgments

We gratefully acknowledge Dr Bradley Foerster and Suzanne Murphy for their kind assistance in the preparation of this manuscript.

References

[1] Bagley Flanders AE, Croul SE. Spine trauma. In: Atlas SW, editor. Magnetic resonance imaging of the brain and spine. 3rd edition. Philadelphia: Lippincott, Williams and Wilkins; 2002. p. 1769–824.

[2] Hill MW, Dean SA. Head injury and facial injury: is there an increased risk of cervical spine injury? J Trauma 1993;34:549–54.

[3] Pope AM, Tarlov AR. Disability in America: toward a national agenda for prevention. Washington, DC: National Academy Press; 1991.

[4] Riggins RS, Kraus JF. The risk of neurological damage with fractures of the vertebrae. J Trauma 1997;17:126–30.

[5] Castellano V, Bocconi FL. Injuries of the cervical spine with spinal cord involvement (myelic fractures): statistical considerations. Bull Hosp Jt Dis Orthop Inst 1970;31:188–98.

[6] Rogers WA. Fractures and dislocations of the cervical spine; an end-result study. J Bone Joint Surg Am 1957;39:341–51.

[7] Pollack CV, Hendey GW, Martin DR, et al. Use of flexion-extension radiographs of the cervical spine in blunt trauma. Ann Emerg Med 2001; 38(1):8–11.

[8] Insko EK, Gracias VH, Gupta R, et al. Utility of flexion and extension radiographs of the cervical spine in the acute evaluation of blunt trauma. J Trauma 2002;53(3):426–9.

[9] Gebhard JS, Donaldson DH, Brown CW. Soft-tissue injuries of the cervical spine. Orthop Rev 1994;23(Suppl):9–17.

[10] Hoffman JR, Mower WR, Wolfson AB, et al. Validity of a set of clinical criteria to rule out injury to the cervical spine in patients with blunt trauma. National Emergency X-radiography Utilization Study group. N Engl J Med 2000;343: 94–9.

[11] Stiell IG, Wells GA, Vandemheen KL, et al. The Canadian C-spine rule for radiography in alert and stable trauma patients. JAMA 2001;286: 1841–8.

[12] Frankel HL, Rozycki GS, Ochsner MG, et al. Indications of obtaining surveillance thoracic and lumbar spine radiographs. J Trauma 1994;37: 673–6.

[13] Widder S, Doig C, Burrowes P, et al. Prospective evaluation of computed tomographic scanning for spinal clearance of obtunded trauma patients: preliminary results. J Trauma 2004;56: 1179–84.

[14] Blackmore CC, Ramsey SD, Mann FA, et al. Cervical spine screening with CT in trauma patients: a cost effectiveness analysis. Radiology 1999;212: 117–25.

[15] Brandt MM, Wahl WL, Yeom K, et al. Computed tomographic scanning reduces costs and time of complete spine evaluation. J Trauma 2004;56: 1022–8.

[16] Tins BJ, Cessar-Pullicino VN. Imaging of acute cervical spine injuries: review and outlook. Clin Radiol 2004;59:865–80.

[17] Blackmore CC, Mann FA, Wilson AJ. Helical CT in the primary trauma evaluation of the cervical spine: an evidence based approach. Skeletal Radiol 2000;29:632–9.

[18] Nunez DB, Quencer RM. The role of helical CT in the assessment of cervical spine injuries. AJR Am J Roentgenol 1998;171:951–7.

[19] Nunez DB, Zuluaga A, Fuentes Bernardo DA, et al. Cervical spine trauma; how much do we learn by routinely using helical CT? Radiographics 1996;16:1307–18.

[20] Diaz JJ Jr, Gillman C, Morris JA Jr, et al. Are five-view plain films of the cervical spine unreliable? A prospective evaluation in blunt trauma in patients with altered mental status. J Trauma 2003;55:658–63.

[21] Griffen MM, Frykberg ER, Kerwin AJ, et al. Radiographic clearance of blunt cervical spine injury: plain radiograph or computed tomography scan? J Trauma 2003;55:222–6.

[22] Holmes JF, Mirvis SE, Panacek EA, et al. For the NEXUS Group. Variability in computed tomography and magnetic resonance imaging in patients with cervical spine injuries. J Trauma 2002;53: 524–9.

[23] Kligman M, Vasili C, Roffman M. The role of computed tomography in cervical spine injury due to diving. Arch Orthop Trauma Surg 2001; 121:139–41.

[24] Schenarts PJ, Diaz J, Kaiser C, et al. Prospective comparison of admission computed tomographic scan and plain films of the upper cervical spine in trauma patients with altered mental status. J Trauma 2001;51:663–8.

[25] Berne JD, Velmahos GC, El Tawil Q, et al. Value of complete cervical helical computed tomographic scanning in identifying cervical spine injury in the unevaluable blunt trauma patient with multiple injuries: a prospective study. J Trauma 1999;47:896–902.

[26] Woodring JH, Lee C. The role and limitations of computed tomography scanning in the evaluation of cervical trauma. J Trauma 1992;33(5): 698–708.

[27] Flanders AE, Schaefer DM, Doan HT, et al. Acute cervical spine trauma; correlation of MR imaging findings with degree of neurological deficit. Radiology 1990;177:25–33.

[28] Sliker CW, Mirvis SE, Shanmuganathan K. Assessing cervical spine stability in obtunded blunt trauma patients; review of medical literature. Radiology 2005;234:733–9.

[29] Wilmink JT. MR imaging of the spine: trauma and degenerative disease. Eur Radiol 1999;9(7): 1259–66.

[30] Smith AS, Hurst GC, Duerk JI, et al. MR of ballistic materials: imaging artifacts and potential hazards. AJNR Am J Neuroradiol 1991;12: 567–72.

[31] Teitelbaum GP, Yee CA, Van Horn DD, et al. Metallic ballistic fragments: MR imaging safety and artifacts. Radiology 1990;175:855–9.

[32] Smugar SS, Schweitzer ME, Hume E. MRI in patients with intraspinal bullets. J Magn Reson Imaging 1999;9:151–3.

[33] Hoffman JR, Wolfson AB, Todd K, et al. Selective cervical spine radiography in blunt trauma: methodology of the National Emergency X-Radiography Utilization Study (NEXUS). Ann Emerg Med 1998;34(4):461–9.

[34] Stiell IG, Clement CM, McKnight RD, et al. The Canadian C-spine rule versus the NEXUS low-risk criteria in patients with trauma. N Engl J Med 2003;349(26):2510–8.

[35] White A III, Panjabi M. Clinical biomechanics of spine. 2nd edition. Philadelphia: JB Lippincott; 1990. p. 722.

[36] Holdsworth H. Fractures, dislocations and fractures-dislocations of the spine. J Bone Joint Surg Br 1963;45:6–20.

[37] Denis F. Three-column spine and its significance in classification of acute thoracolumbar spine injuries. Spine 1983;8:817–32.

[38] Louis R. Spinal stability as defined by three-column spine concept. Anat Clin 1985;7:33–42.

[39] Goldberg W, Mueller C, Panacek E, et al. Distribution and patterns of blunt traumatic cervical spine injury. Ann Emerg Med 2001;38(1):17–21.

[40] Cirak B, Ziegfeld S, Knight VM, et al. Spinal injuries in children. J Pediatr Surg 2004;39(4):607–12.

[41] Bensch FV, Kiuru MJ, Koivikko MP, et al. Spine fractures in falling accidents: analysis of multidetector CT findings. Eur Radiol 2004;14(4):618–24.

[42] McCall T, Fassett D, Brockmeyer D. Cervical spin trauma in children: a review. Neurosurg Focus 2006;20(2):1–8.

[43] Effendi B, Roy D, Cornish B, et al. Fractures of the ring of the axis: a classification based on the analysis of 131 cases. J Bone Joint Surg Br 1981;63:319–27.

[44] Cusick JF, Yoganandan N. Biomechanics of the cervical spine 4: major injuries. Clin Biomech (Bristol, Avon) 2002;17:1–20.

[45] Spitzer WO, Skovron ML, Salmi RS, et al. Scientific monograph of the Quebec Task Force on whiplash-associated disorders: redefining "whiplash" and its management. Spine 1995;20:1S–73S.

[46] Ronnen HR, de Korte PJ, Brink PR, et al. Acute whiplash injury: is there a role for MR imaging?—a prospective study of 100 patients. Radiology 1996;201:93–6.

[47] Borchgrevink G, Smevik O, Haave I, et al. MRI of the cerebrum and cervical column within two weeks after whiplash neck sprain injury. Injury 1997;28:351–5.

[48] Pettersson K, Hildingsson C, Toolanen G, et al. Disc pathology after whiplash injury; a prospective magnetic resonance imaging and clinical investigation. Spine 1997;22:283–7.

[49] Rodriquez AA, Barr KP, Burns SP. Whiplash: pathophysiology, diagnosis, treatment and prognosis. Muscle Nerve 2004;29:768–81.

[50] Ovadia D, Steinberg EI, Nissan M, et al. Whiplash injury: a retrospective study on patients seeking compensation. Injury 2002;33:569–73.

[51] Jonsson H, Cesarini K, Sahlstedt B, et al. Findings and outcome in whiplash-type neck distortions. Spine 1994;19:2733–43.

[52] Rogers LF. The roentgenographic appearances of transverse or chance fractures of the spine: the seat belt fracture. AJR Am J Roentgenol 1971; 111:844–9.

[53] Gertzbein SD. Scoliosis Research Society: multicenter spine fracture study. Spine 1992;17:528–40.

[54] Dai LY. Imaging diagnosis of thoracolumbar burst fractures. Chin Med Sci J 2004;19(2):142–4.

[55] Ballock RT, Mackersie R, Abitbol JJ, et al. Can burst fracture be predicted from plain radiographs? J Bone Joint Surg Br 1992;74:147–50.

[56] Burney R, Maio RF, Maynard F, et al. Incidence, characteristics and outcome of spinal cord injury at trauma centers in North America. Arch Surg 1993;128(5):596–9.

[57] McDonald JW, Sadowsky C. Spinal cord injury. Lancet 2002;359(9304):417–25.

[58] Beattie MS, Farooqui AA, Bresnahan JC. Review of current evidence for apoptosis after spinal cord injury. J Neurotrauma 2000;17:915–26.

[59] Cohen ME, Sheehan TP, Herbison GJ. Content validity and reliability of the International Standards for Neurological Classification of Spinal Cord Injury. Topics Spine Cord Injury Rehabil 1996;4:15–31.

[60] Maynard FM Jr, Bracken MB, Creasey G, et al. International standards for neurological and functional classification of spinal cord injury: American Spinal Injury Association. Spinal Cord 1997;35:266–74.

[61] Waters RL, Adkins RH, Yakura JS, et al. Motor and sensory recovery following incomplete tetraplegia. Arch Phys Med Rehabil 1994;75:306–11.

[62] Marino RJ, Ditunno JF Jr, Donovan WH, et al. Neurologic recovery after traumatic spinal cord injury. Data from the model spinal cord systems. Arch Phys Med Rehabil 1999;80:1391–6.

[63] Van Goethem JWM, Maes M, Özsarlak Ö, et al. Imaging of the spinal trauma. Eur Radiol 2005; 15:582–90.

[64] Yue JJ, Lawrence BD, Sutton KM, et al. Complete cervical intervertebral disc extrusion with spinal cord injury in the absence of facet dislocation: a case report. Spine 2004;29(9):181–4.

[65] Diaz JJ, Aulino JM, Collier B, et al. The early work-up for isolated ligamentous injury of the cervical spine; does computed tomography scan have a role. J Trauma 2005;59:897–904.

[66] Platzer P, Jaindl M, Thalhammar G, et al. Clearing the cervical spine in critically injured patients: a comprehensive C-spine protocol to avoid unnecessary delays in diagnosis. Eur Spine J 2006;15(12):1801–10.

[67] Weisskopf M, Bail H, Mack M, et al. Value of MRI in traumatic disco-ligament instability of the lower cervical spine. Unfallchirurg 1999; 102(12):942–8 [in German].

[68] Song J, Mizuno J, Inoue T, et al. Clinical evaluation of traumatic central cord syndrome: emphasis on clinical significance of prevertebral hyperintensity, cord compression, and intramedullary high-signal intensity on magnetic resonance imaging. Surg Neurol 2006;65:117–23.

[69] Chiau WC, Haan JM, Cushing BM, et al. Ligamentous injuries of the cervical spine in unreliable blunt trauma patients: incidence, evaluation, and outcome. J Trauma 2001;50(3):457–63.

[70] Burke DC. Traumatic spinal paralysis in children. Paraplegia 1974;11:268–76.

[71] Dula DJ. Trauma to the cervical spine. JACEP 1979;8:504–7.

[72] Hubbard DD. Injuries of the spine in children and adolescents. Clin Orthop Relat Res 1974; 100:56–65.

[73] Melzak J. Paraplegia among children. Lancet 1969;2:45–8.

[74] Henrys P, Lyne ED, Lifton C, et al. Clinical review of cervical spine injuries in children. Clin Orthop Relat Res 1977;129:172–6.

[75] Ruge JR, Sinson GP, McLong DG, et al. Pediatric spinal injury: the very young. J Neurosurg 1988; 68:25–30.

[76] Hadley MN, Zabramski JM, Browner CM, et al. Pediatric spinal trauma. Review of 122 cases of spinal cord or vertebral column injuries. J Neurosurg 1988;68:18–24.

[77] Kewalramani LS, Kraus JF, Sterling HM. Acute spinal-cord lesions in a pediatric population: epidemiological and clinical features. Paraplegia 1980;18:206–19.

[78] Pang D, Wilberger JE Jr. Spinal cord injury without radiographic abnormalities in children. J Neurosurg 1982;57:114–29.

[79] Imhof H, Fuchsjäger M. Traumatic injuries: imaging of spinal injuries. Eur Radiol 2002;12: 1262–72.

[80] Potter K, Saifuddin A. Pictorial review: MRI of chronic spinal cord injury. Br J Radiol 2003; 76(905):347–52.

ELSEVIER
SAUNDERS

NEUROIMAGING
CLINICS
OF NORTH AMERICA

Neuroimag Clin N Am 17 (2007) 87–103

Degenerative Disease of the Spine

Massimo Gallucci, MD[a],*, Nicola Limbucci, MD[a],
Amalia Paonessa, MD[b], Alessandra Splendiani, MD[a]

- Physiopathology
- Imaging methods: indications
  and techniques
- Radiologic semiotic

- *Bone structures*
- *Intervertebral discs*
- References

Degenerative disease of the spine is a definition that includes a wide spectrum of degenerative abnormalities. Degeneration involves bony structures and the intervertebral disc, although many aspects of spine degeneration are strictly linked because the main common pathogenic factor is identified in chronic overload. During life the spine undergoes continuous changes as a response to physiologic axial load. These age-related changes are similar to pathologic degenerative changes and are a common asymptomatic finding in adults and elderly persons. A mild degree of degenerative changes is paraphysiologic and should be considered pathologic only if abnormalities determine symptoms. Imaging allows complete evaluation of static and dynamic factors related to degenerative disease of the spine and is useful in diagnosing the different aspects of spine degeneration.

Physiopathology

The causes of age-related and pathologic spine degenerative changes are multiple: traumatic, metabolic, toxic, genetic, vascular, and infectious. Trauma is the main pathologic factor, however, including chronic overload, chronic multitraumatism, and sequelae of acute trauma [1,2]. The concept of chronic duration trauma has the highest

relevance, because degenerative disease of the spine is actually considered the consequence of overuse injury. Abnormal stresses, not sufficient to cause fracture, can be responsible for bone and disc damage if applied for long period. In most cases, the alterations involve the disc and the vertebral body because of the morphologic-functional relationship between these structures [3].

The distribution of axial load is responsible for the typical localization of spine degeneration. C5-6 and C6-7 levels are involved in most cases, because they are the sites of lordosis inversion. In the dorsal spine degeneration is rare, because this tract is less mobile and less involved in dynamic load. In the lumbosacral tract the most frequently degenerated levels are L4-5 and L5-S1, because they are the sites of the highest dynamic and static load [1,2,4]. The functional integrity of spinal curves is involved in degenerative changes. Spinal curves allow optimal redistribution of axial load. When curves are preserved, the spine is 30 times more elastic than a straight structure. If correct spine alignment is lost, an asymmetrical load distribution may cause focal or diffuse spine degeneration.

Because of overlap of imaging findings in age-related changes and degenerative changes, it is usually difficult to define whether abnormalities are

[a] Department of Radiology, University of L'Aquila, S. Salvatore Hospital, Via Vetoio, Loc. Coppito, 67100 L'Aquila, Italy
[b] Department of Neuroradiology, Loreto Nuovo Hospital, Naples, Italy
* Corresponding author.
E-mail address: massimo.gallucci@cc.univaq.it (M. Gallucci).

doi:10.1016/j.nic.2007.01.002

paraphysiologic or pathologic. Evaluation of the presence of congruous symptoms and the severity of abnormalities is mandatory for a correct diagnosis [2,5,6].

Progressive involution of the spinal structures begins after the second decade and invariably determines some degree of vertebral and discal degeneration. The first sign of degeneration is the appearance of intranuclear clefts, which are virtually present in 100% of discs after 40 years [7]. Frequently in the adult population asymptomatic disc dehydration and radial fissures can be observed; in elderly persons a slight degree of osteochondrosis and other bony degenerative changes is normal and is considered paraphysiologic. The main difference between people with asymptomatic age-related changes and degenerative abnormalities is the presence of an abnormal axial load distribution in patients with degeneration. Overuse injuries develop pathologically at a younger age in these people than in the healthy elderly population [6].

Imaging methods: indications and techniques

Imaging plays an important role in the evaluation of degenerative spine. Indication for radiologic examination and technique should be evaluated in every case [8]. When a patient complains of typical back or monoradicular pain, there is no statistical risk in waiting 4 to 6 weeks before performing any radiologic examination. In many cases there is a high possibility of spontaneous pain regression, especially in cases of small acute herniations and extraspinal disorders, such as neuritis and muscular or insertional inflammation. Patients with a history of neoplasm, atypical pain, neurologic deficit, and other local or systemic symptoms should be evaluated earlier.

Plain films still play an important role in evaluation of the spine, because the examination is inexpensive and promptly available and gives a wide panoramic view of the spine. Direct information about bony structures can be obtained, and functional information about misalignment and vertebral stability can be obtained with upright dynamic films in flexion-extension and lateral bending [9].

When findings on plain films do not give sufficient explanation of symptoms, CT or MRI should be performed. If bony abnormalities are diagnosed or highly suspected, CT may be performed for a more complete evaluation. In elderly patients with low back pain or sciatica it is even more commonly accepted as a valid alternative to MRI [10].

Myelography is rarely performed and reserved for patients with contraindications to MRI or in whom subtle instability is suspected but not confirmed by other examinations. Discography is also reserved for selected patients before some interventional procedures or when the diagnosis of discogenic pain must be confirmed.

For accurate instability evaluation, plain films usually do not offer complete information. The main cause is absent direct visualization of cerebrospinal fluid and nervous structures. Weight-bearing CT and MRI are imaging alternatives. An axial loader is a hydraulic compressor that is placed below a patient's feet and over the shoulders to apply a variable axial load on the spine. The device can be used with CT or MRI, and it simulates static mechanical forces acting on the spine in the upright position [11]. More recently, dedicated MRI units that allow examination with the patient in the upright position have been realized. These systems have the advantage of determining axial load by gravity, a patient's weight, and spine morphology without artificial simulation [12,13]. With the same units, cervical dynamic flexion-extension evaluation is possible.

Radiologic semiotic

Bone structures

Vertebral osteochondrosis

Vertebral endplates bone marrow alterations are a common finding in patients with degenerative spine disease and are strictly associated with disc degeneration. To describe these changes, in 1985, Resnick [2] introduced the concept of vertebral osteochondrosis. This concept is considered an evolutionary process characterized by six phases: (1) disc thinning and hyaline degeneration, (2) chondral microfractures, (3) chondroblastic activation, (4) subchondral reactive neovascularization, (5) bony trabeculae demineralization, and (6) osteosclerosis.

Osteochondrosis is present in 19% of asymptomatic people [14]. It has been found in 50% of people who complain of low-back pain, however [15]. Reversible symptoms can be determined by acute inflammation in type I osteochondrosis, whereas other types are usually asymptomatic. Osteochondrosis is more frequent at levels at which the axial load is higher, such as L4-5 and L5-S1. The relationship with degenerative disc disease is probably caused by multiple factors, including common biomechanical factors, raised mechanical stresses on the endplates induced by disc dehydration, and disc metabolism changes. Other theories consider that the disc is an avascular structure supplied by diffusion from endplate cartilage; therefore, endplate alterations can induce disc trophism defects.

In 1988, Modic et al. [16] proposed a simple classification of vertebral osteochondrosis based on pathologic and imaging aspects. Modic type I (vascular pattern) is a discovertebritis or aseptic spondylodiscitis with bone inflammatory reaction associated with disc degeneration. In this phase, MRI signal of the endplates is low on T1-weighted and high on T2-weighted sequences (Fig. 1). Modic type I can be reversible or can progress [17]. Modic type II (fatty pattern) is characterized by subchondral bone marrow changes with fatty marrow prevalence and demineralization. Endplate MRI signal is high on T1- and T2-weighted sequences (Fig. 2). Modic type III (sclerotic pattern) is the final subchondral osteosclerotic evolution and is characterized by low signal on T1- and T2-weighted sequences (Fig. 3). In this last case, plain films and CT clearly show endplate sclerosis. In almost all cases of vertebral osteochondrosis, MRI shows clear signs of disc degeneration. Sometimes more types are simultaneously found at the same level. In advanced cases, marginal traction osteophytes are frequently found. With MRI, differentiation between Modic types is usually possible. Diagnostic problems can be encountered in differential diagnosis between type I and infectious spondilodiscitis, however. In this case, gadolinium administration is useful, because in type I osteochondrosis disc enhancement is usually absent. In both cases subchondral enhancement can be registered.

Spondylosis

The most typical consequence of age- or load-related degeneration of the vertebral bodies is spondylosis deformans [2]. Spondylosis is found in 60% of women and 80% of men after the age of 50. In elderly people some degree of spondylosis is almost always found and can be considered paraphysiologic. When degenerative alterations are severe or symptomatic, they should be considered pathologic.

The classic sign of spondylosis is osteophytosis. Osteophytes are bony spurs that originate on the anterolateral aspect of the vertebral bodies a few millimeters from the margins of the disc space. They result from weakening and radial degeneration of the fibers of the annulus, with increased vertebral mobility and traction on Sharpey's fibers determining subsequent osteogenic stimulation. Osteophytes usually follow Sharpey's fibers. At the beginning they have a triangular shape and extend on the horizontal plane; in the more advanced phase they become hooked and grow vertically. Sometimes osteophytes develop on both sites of a disc space and grow until they fuse together to form a "bridge osteophyte" [2]. Although the most frequent site of osteophytosis is the anterolateral aspect of the vertebra, posterior osteophytes have higher clinical significance because of the possible compression of neural structures. Posterior osteophytes more frequently accompany osteophytes associated with osteochondrosis, microinstability, and disc degeneration. They are characterized by a bulky triangular shape and have a marginal location [6].

Plain films are adequate for the diagnosis of spondylosis and are helpful for the differential diagnosis between osteophytosis and other bony excrescences with different origin (Fig. 3A). CT and MRI can show the osteophytes, but they are useful for identifying other associated degenerative changes and establishing the relationship between bone and neural structures (Fig. 3B) [7,10].

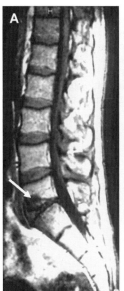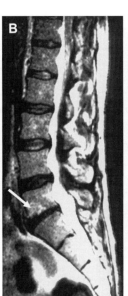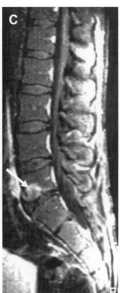

Fig. 1. Modic type I. (*A*) Hypointense area is demonstrated involving the lower endplate of L5 (*arrow*) on sagittal T1-weighted SE MRI. (*B, C*) Corresponding hyperintensity is seen on Fast Spin-Echo T2-weighted MR (*B*) and short-tau inversion-recovery (STIR) (*C*) images.

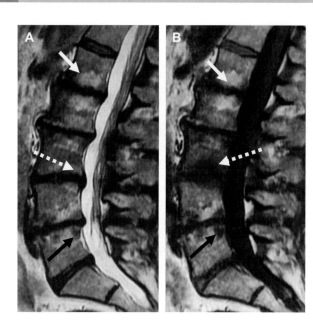

Fig. 2. Modic type II and III. (*A, B*) The end-plates at L1-2 level (*white arrow*) show hyperintensity on T1- (*A*) and T2-weighted (*B*) sequences because of type II osteochondrosis. At L3-4 (*dotted arrow*), mild type I osteochondrosis is present. At L4-5, the signal is inhomogeneous, with evidence of type III osteochondrosis in the posterior aspect of the endplates (*black arrow*).

Schmorl's node is a common sign of spinal degeneration that is often included in the spectrum of spondylosis, although it has a distinct pathogenesis. A Schmorl's node is a herniation of the intervertebral disc through the endplate in the vertebral body and is a frequent incidental finding. Schmorl's nodes are usually asymptomatic; however, in the acute phase they can determine temporary back pain. Imaging shows a central defect of the upper endplate of the vertebral body, often with a clear sclerotic rim. MRI best depicts the relationship between the herniated material and the disc, which is often dehydrated. Acute nodes can be hyperintense on T2-weighted sequences and can enhance after gadolinium administration.

Degenerative changes of the cervical spine typically involve the uncovertebral processes with formation of posterior osteophytes. Associated abnormalities are disc height decrease and disc bulging or protrusion. Plain films are useful for the evaluation of cervical uncoarthrosis; the examination should be completed with oblique projections because osteophytes often determine stenosis of the neural foramina and otherwise could be missed (Fig. 4). MRI is required to identify disc herniations that can determine spinal canal

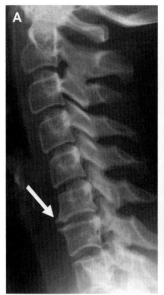
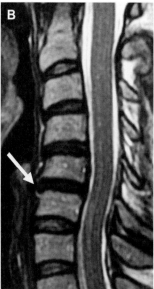

Fig. 3. Spondylosis. (*A*) Plain film in a patient with cervical spondylosis clearly shows anterior osteophytes with endplate sclerosis and disc space narrowing (*arrow*). (*B*) Sagittal T2-weighted MRI of a different patient shows submarginal osteophytes with hooked shape (*arrow*) and disc dehydration.

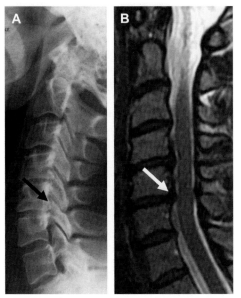

Fig. 4. Cervical osteoarthritis involving the uncinate processes. (*A*) Plain film shows multiple posterior osteophytes (*arrow*). (*B*) With MRI, osteophytes are less visible, but bulging and dehydrated discs in C4-5 and C5-6 are evident.

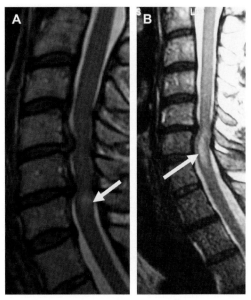

Fig. 5. Cervical myelopathy. (*A*) Sagittal T2-weighted Fast Spin-Echo MRI clearly shows a hyperintense focal area, which suggests myelopathy, with corresponding disc herniations determining central canal stenosis. (*B*) Sagittal T2-weighted Fast Spin-Echo MRI in another patient shows a wide hyperintense area (*arrow*) below a cervical canal stenosis, which suggests associated ischemic changes in the spinal cord.

stenosis and possible compressive myelopathy (Fig. 5).

Facet joints

Facet joints are frequently involved in osteoarthritis. The typical imaging findings are joint space narrowing, subchondral sclerosis and cysts, osteophytosis, ligament thickening, intra-articular vacuum and joint fluid. Osteophytes can involve the whole facet that appears hypertrophic; however, they more often involve the articular surface of the superior facet of the lower vertebra, because the inferior is covered by the ligamentum flavum. Plain films can show the presence of degenerative changes; however, the anatomic complexity of this region requires CT or MRI for a complete evaluation of the degenerative process. Severe facet osteoarthritis can determine lateral recess and neural foramen stenosis; less frequently, canal stenosis can be observed. CT is more accurate for determining bony abnormalities, but MRI more clearly shows neural structures and soft tissues (Fig. 6).

Facet joint osteoarthritis often leads to vertebral instability because of sagittal orientation of the articular rim and degenerative weakening of the capsule and the periarticular structures [18]. Abnormal orientation of the articular rim can be sometimes congenital and rarely asymmetric. In these cases facet joint osteoarthritis and instability develop earlier. Facet instability leads to anterior subluxation of the inferior facet of the upper vertebra or degenerative spondylolisthesis. Weight-bearing MRI can be useful in selected cases to diagnose facet joint instability, which appears as joint space widening and anterior slippage of the lower facet. Weight-bearing MRI also can show increased thickening of the ligamentum flavum during axial load caused by ligament laxity. This process can determine appearance of a stenosis only during axial loading [13]. The role of facet joints in back pain is often difficult to assess, because symptoms can be unspecific and imaging findings of degeneration are common [19]. In selected cases, nerve block or facet joint steroid and anesthetic injections are useful for diagnostic and therapeutic purposes, because they reduce pain for patients who have facet syndrome [20].

Rarely, patients with hyperlordosis and severe degenerative changes of the facet joints can develop Baastrup disease. This condition is characterized by interspinosus contact, with resulting inflammatory reaction and possible formation of pseudoarticulation.

Sometimes facet joint degeneration is complicated by synovial cysts. These formations originate from the joint and can keep or lose the connection with the joint. When they develop on the

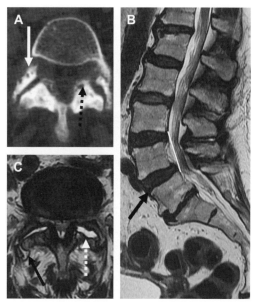

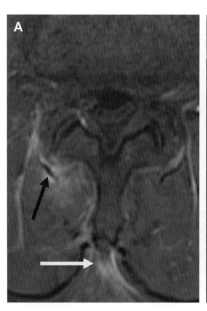

Fig. 6. Facet joints osteoarthritis. (*A*) On CT subchondral sclerosis, geodes and widening of the joint rim (*white arrow*) are demonstrated. Calcification of the ligamenta flava also is evident (*dotted black arrow*). (*B*) On MRI, bone abnormalities are less clear but the examination is more accurate for visualization of ligament thickening and articular space widening. Lateral stenosis is well demonstrated. Note right posterior synovial cyst (*black arrow*). (*C*) Sagittal Fast Spin-Echo T2-weighted sequence shows L4 low-grade spondylolisthesis. Note also anterior osteophytes in L5-S1.

intracanalicular side of a joint, they can have compressive effects (Fig. 6B). Cysts can contain synovial serous fluid, more gelatinous material, air, or blood. The diagnosis and the connection with the joint can be confirmed by percutaneous CT or fluoroscopic-guided aspiration. After aspiration, the cyst can be filled with steroid and anesthetic and can be broken for curative purposes.

Facet joint synovitis has been recognized as a possible cause of facet syndrome. Typical MRI findings are intra-articular or pericapsular high signal on T2-weighted sequences and enhancement after contrast agent administration (Fig. 7) [7].

Spondylolysis and spondylolisthesis

Six types of spondylolysis have been defined: dysplastic, isthmic, traumatic, pathologic, iatrogenic, and degenerative (pseudospondylolysis). The most common kind of lumbar spondylolysis is the isthmic type, which is a typical pathologic condition of children, adolescents, and young adults. Isthmic spondylolysis can be defined as a defect of the pars interarticularis of the vertebra and it is considered a fatigue fracture produced by abnormal mechanical stresses on an otherwise normal bone. Spondylolysis is initiated by repetitive direct microtraumas, repeated contraction of agonist and antagonist muscles, and mechanical load of the body weight. These factors induce a stress response in the bone. The most common site of spondylolysis is L5 (81%) followed by L4 (14%). The prevalence of spondylolysis in the general asymptomatic population is approximately 3% to 7%, but it is higher in people who participate in sports activity [21,22].

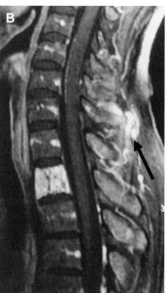

Fig. 7. Soft tissues abnormalities. (*A*) Fat saturated Fast Spin-Echo T1-weighted MRI after contrast administration shows abnormal enhancement of the interspinous ligament (*white arrow*) and the pericapsular tissues of right facet joint (*black arrow*). (*B*) In another patient, enhancement of the cervical interspinous ligament (*arrow*) is observed. Note an asymptomatic vertebral hemangioma.

Plain films are useful for diagnosing spondylolysis: a lateral view often allows identifying the isthmic lysis as a defect of the pars interarticularis with sclerotic borders, but the examination should be completed by 45° oblique view. On this projection, spondylolysis can be recognized for the classic sign of the "Scottish terrier's collar." Single-photon emission CT is sensitive for the detection of spondylolysis in the acute phase; older or asymptomatic lesions can be silent because of the absence of active bone reaction. CT is accurate for the detection of lysis, which appears as transverse isthmic fracture with irregular rim and sclerosis (Fig. 8A) [21]. The examination should be performed with a reverse gantry angle (15%–25%) parallel to the axis of the isthmus; otherwise, differentiation between the lysis and normal facet joints can be difficult [23]. MRI is less sensitive and less accurate than CT; lysis can be distinguished on MRI as an interruption of the normal bony signal (Fig. 8B).

Spondylolysis often leads to spondylolisthesis, which is defined as anterior or posterior slippage of a vertebral body. In the elderly population, spondylolisthesis is frequent (approximately 4%) and is usually not related to spondylolysis but to severe degeneration of the interapophyseal joints. The typical sites of degenerative spondylolisthesis are L3-4 and L4-5 because of the more sagittal orientation of the joints. Anterior spondylolisthesis can be classified in four grades according to Meyerding's classification. Degenerative spondylolisthesis is usually grade I (slippage below 25%). Posterior spondylolisthesis is a posterior subluxation of the body that is usually associated with facet joints and disc degeneration. This alteration is more frequent at more mobile spine segments, such as the cervical tract and upper lumbar levels. If spondylolisthesis is caused by isthmic lysis, the anterior slippage causes widening of the vertebral canal. Conversely, when spondylolisthesis has a degenerative origin the canal undergoes anteroposterior narrowing because of slippage of the posterior vertebral arch and facet hypertrophy [18].

Upright plain films are necessary for a correct diagnosis and grading of spondylolisthesis. Dynamic radiographs in hyperflexion, hyperextension, and lateral bending are useful for evaluating associated vertebral instability, which is characterized by loss of alignment of one of more vertebral lines (Fig. 9). Radiographic signs of instability obtained with dynamic films are evidence of anterior or posterior vertebral slippage during motion or load, pedicle length variations, neural foramina narrowing, and loss of intervertebral disc height. Other associated signs are intradiscal vacuum and traction osteophytes. Conventional MRI can show spondylolisthesis, but its value is limited for functional information. MRI often shows "pseudobulging," which usually occurs at the level of the lysis, and narrowing of the neural foramina (Fig. 10). Axial loaded CT and MRI or upright MRI can provide functional information about vertebral stability and spine response to physiologic load conditions (Fig. 11) [24].

Degenerative stenosis

Degenerative changes can determine spinal stenosis, including central canal stenosis, lateral recess stenosis, and foraminal stenosis. Spinal stenosis is classified as congenital, acquired, or mixed. Congenital stenosis is more frequent in the lumbar tract. It can be part of a skeletal syndrome (eg, Morquio's sign, achondroplasia, Down syndrome) or be idiopathic. The latter condition is characterized by shortness and thickness of the pedicles, shortness of laminae, or sagittal orientation of facet joints. Acquired stenosis is usually caused by degenerative bony and discal changes. They usually involve the cervical and lumbar tracts, whereas the thoracic spine is rarely

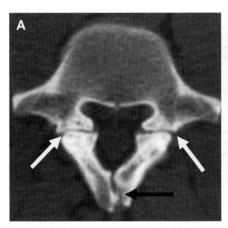
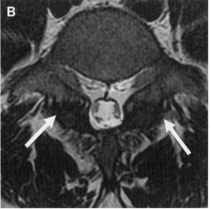

Fig. 8. Lythic spondylolysis of L5. (*A*) CT clearly depicts the bilateral lysis of the pars interarticularis (*white arrows*). (*B*) MRI findings are more subtle. Note posterior median schisis (*black arrow*).

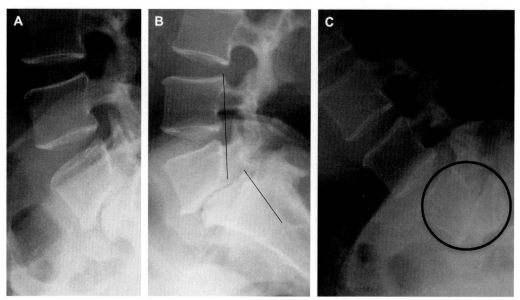

Fig. 9. Degenerative spondylolisthesis. (*A–C*) Dynamic radiographs: neutral (*A*), during extension (*B*), and flexion (*C*). Note increase of vertebral slippages during flexion (*C*).

affected. Mixed stenoses are caused by degenerative abnormalities in patients with a constitutionally narrow spinal canal [1].

The definition of central stenosis is subjective, although many studies tried to define stenosis on the basis of quantitative parameters. At the cervical level, an indicative value of early stenosis is a sagittal canal diameter <14 mm between C4 and C7. If the anteroposterior diameter is <11 mm, the patient

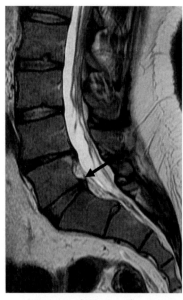

Fig. 10. Pseudobulging. Patient with minimal spondylolisthesis of L5 with posterior exposure of the disc demonstrated on sagittal T2-weighted MRI (*arrow*).

usually experiences neurologic symptoms. Alternatively, stenosis should be considered if the ratio between canal sagittal diameter and body sagittal diameter is <0.8 mm. In the lumbar spine, normal median sagittal diameter is >15 mm. Moderate stenosis is established if the diameter is between 14 and 10 mm; severe stenosis is established if the diameter is <10 mm. In some cases, the sagittal diameter undergoes a slight narrowing because the transverse diameter can markedly decrease, and interpeduncular diameter should be considered. This diameter usually measures 17 to 19 mm at L1 and 20 to 23 mm at L5. Although measurement of canal diameters can be useful, its correlation with symptoms is low. Imaging evaluation is mainly based on subjective evaluation of canal morphology and the relationship between the dimensions of the containing and the contained structures.

All aspects of degenerative spinal disease contribute to spinal stenosis, and in most cases more factors are simultaneously present and variously combined. Disc bulging or herniations, spondylosis deformans, osteochondrosis with traction osteophytes, facet joint osteoarthritis (see Fig. 6), ligamentum flavum thickening, asymmetric facet joint orientation (Fig. 12), and ligament calcifications can determine canalicular stenosis because of direct compression. Stenosis can be more evident in orthostatis when dynamic factors contribute to its genesis. This condition happens in patients with significant vertebral instability or spondylolisthesis [18].

Lateral recess stenosis is usually caused by hypertrophy and osteophytosis of the superior articular

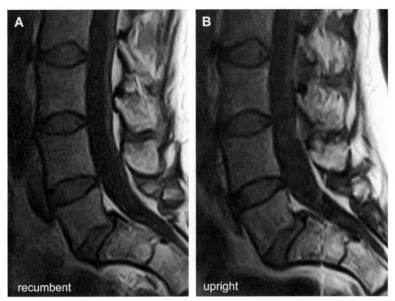

Fig. 11. Spondylolisthesis. (*A, B*) MR examination performed in recumbent (*A*) and upright (*B*) positions with a dedicated low field unit. At baseline, low-grade L5 spondylolisthesis is evident; in upright position the abnormality appears more severe.

facet; less frequently the stenosis is caused by vertebral body osteophytosis or other degenerative changes. The stenosis can be isolated but usually involves the central part of the canal. The normal sagittal diameter of the lateral recess is >5 mm; when this space is <4 mm the recess is considered stenotic [7].

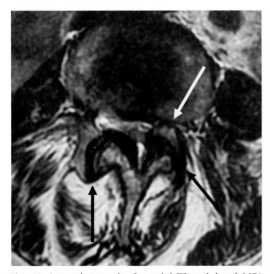

Fig. 12. Lateral stenosis. On axial T2-weighted MRI, asymmetric orientation of the facet joints—with the left one horizontal and the right sagittal—is observed. This morphology induces abnormal facet joint degeneration and lateral recess stenosis. Note atrophy of psoas and spinal muscles.

Foraminal stenosis is more common than lateral recess stenosis. It is usually caused by disc material and marginal osteophytes protruding into the foramen. Another common cause is narrowing of the disc space with subsequent anterosuperior slippage of the superior facet.

The role of imaging in spinal stenosis is to confirm the clinical diagnosis, identify the level of stenosis, establish causes, and guide treatment. Plain films are useful for measuring the diameter of the canal and evaluating bony abnormalities. Cross-sectional imaging is necessary for a complete balance of the entity and causes of spinal stenosis, however. CT is the gold standard for evaluation of bony abnormalities and is accurate for detecting posterior osteophytosis (Fig. 13). The dural sac and the nervous structures are visible and their compression can be assessed. CT is useful for identifying calcifications of the ligamentum flavum and the posterior longitudinal ligament, which can play an important role in the genesis of stenosis, especially at thoracic level [25]. Calcifications can be missed easily by MRI, because degeneration of posterior arch structures is often homogeneously hyperintense because of the presence of marked fibrosis and bone sclerosis. MRI accurately depicts the disc pathology and shows nervous structures more clearly. At the lumbar level the hyperintense signal of cerebrospinal fluid on T2-weighted sequences offers a myelographic effect because of the high contrast resolution between the dural sac and the extradural structures. This effect can be

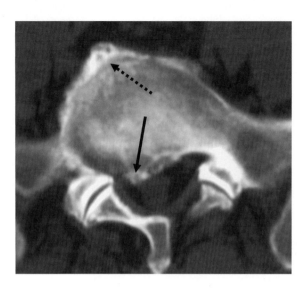

Fig. 13. Spinal stenosis. On CT, a bulky posterior marginal osteophyte (*arrow*) determines narrowing of the central canal and the lateral recess. Note anterolateral osteophyte (*dotted arrow*).

stressed and myelo-MRI can be obtained; however, their clinical usefulness is limited. The best diagnostic sign is the reduction of the dimensions of the dural sac or the spinal cord, with hypertrophy of the surrounding bony and discal structures. Epidural fat is reduced or disappears on axial scan planes. On sagittal T2-weighted sequences, multiple anterior and posterior notches on the dural sac can be observed, the former caused by disc and vertebral body abnormalities and the latter caused by facet joint and ligamentum flavum thickening [25]. Vertebral body osteophytes are usually detected. They are often hypointense, however, and the distinction between osteophytes and the hypointense herniated disc can be difficult to make. In this case gradient echo (GE) T2-weighted sequences are useful because they enhance the intrinsic contrast between the disc (hyperintense) and the osteophyte (hypointense).

A finding sometimes observed in patients with severe lumbar central canal stenosis is so-called "redundant nerve roots," which present as enlarged and swollen aspects of cauda equina nerve roots (Fig. 14). Redundant nerve roots are supposed to be caused by increased cerebrospinal fluid pressure and radicular venous congestion caused by the stenosis. The consequence would be radicular ischemic damage and edema [1]. Constitutional abnormalities that contribute to mixed stenosis are easily detected by imaging and must be reported for their implication on stenosis management (Fig. 15).

In cervical and dorsal stenosis, MRI shows not only spinal degenerative changes but also disappearance of subarachnoid space and narrowing and compression of the spinal cord (see Fig. 5).

MRI is helpful for diagnosing myelopathy, which appears as smooth, hyperintense areas on T2-weighted sequences. Rarely syringomyelic cavities are present. In compressive myelopathy, abnormal areas are usually located at the level of stenosis; however, sometimes they are found below the stenosis (see Fig. 5B). These abnormalities are probably caused by ischemia, because increased cerebrospinal fluid at the stenotic level leads to reduced venous drainage and spinal cord venous congestion, which result in cord ischemic damage.

Dynamic plain films, weight-bearing CT, and MRI have been applied to the study of spinal stenosis [12]. Under axial loading or in an upright position, the stenosis can be more evident because of modifications of the intermetameric relationships induced by increased load, especially in patients with vertebral instability (Fig. 16). In patients with kinetic-dependent instability and stenosis, the alterations can become evident only during weight-bearing or dynamic examination. Longitudinal hypermobility of the facet joints with anterior slippage of the articular processes is responsible for augmented central or lateral stenosis [18], which appears as increased degree of spondylolisthesis and increased protrusion of the articular processes into the canal. Disc herniations are sometimes more pronounced under weight bearing. Ligamenta flava hyperlaxity is another important cause of stenosis. It can appear more severe during weight-bearing examinations because narrowing of disc space determines shortening and thickening of the ligaments. Thanks to high signal of cerebrospinal fluid, myelographic semeiotic can be applied to upright MRI. Narrowing of perimedullary

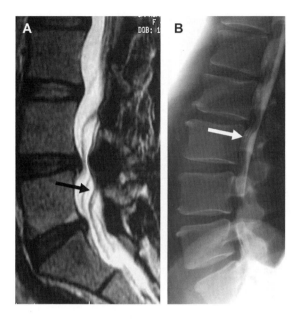

Fig. 14. Redundant nerve roots. (*A*) Fast Spin-Echo T2-weighted MRI shows central stenosis at L4-5 caused by facet joint osteoarthritis and bulging disc. Cauda nerve roots appear thickened and tortuous (*arrow*). (*B*) Myelography of a different patient shows thickened roots (*arrow*).

subarachnoid space and decrease of dural sac diameter during upright and dynamic examinations are important signs of stenosis.

Intervertebral discs

Pathophysiology

Degeneration of intervertebral disc is characterized by dehydration, fissures, bulging, and herniations. Degenerative disc disease is more common in the elderly population; however, acute herniations are frequent in the middle-aged population. Three main pathogenetic mechanisms are involved in degenerative disc disease:

1. Acute trauma, which leads to vertebral instability with alterations of spinal alignment that can accelerate degeneration. This mechanism is frequently related to the discovertebral degeneration observed after an acute cervical trauma.
2. Chronic static and dynamic overload, which causes chronic microtraumas. This is considered

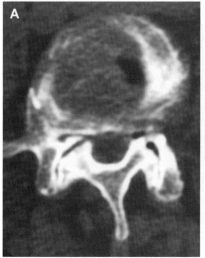
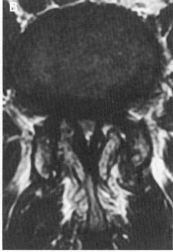

Fig. 15. Mixed stenosis. (*A*) CT scan in central lumbar stenosis induced by slight degenerative changes in a patient with constitutional short pedicles. (*B*) MRI of a different patient with central stenosis promoted by sagittal orientation of the facet joints with anterior subluxation.

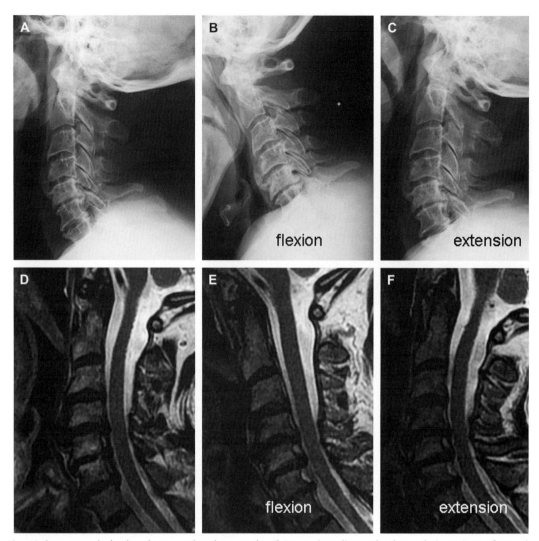

Fig. 16. Severe cervical spine degenerative changes. (*A–C*) Dynamic radiographs show obvious signs of spondylosis and uncoarthrosis, with rigidity of the rachis and signs of instability. (*D–F*) Dynamic MR examination confirms radiographic findings and offers additional information about soft tissues. In this case the diameter of the canal is slightly reduced during flexion-extension, but the spinal cord is not compressed.

the most important factor leading to disc degeneration. It is also proven by the higher prevalence of disc herniations at levels of maximal axial load.

3. Decreased permeability of the endplates, which leads to dysfunction of fibroblasts and chondrocytes, with subsequent alteration of the keratin/chondroitin sulfate ratio. Matrix degeneration determines loss of nucleus pulposus water and consequent rigidity.

Classification and imaging

The first phase of disc degeneration is dehydration of the nucleus pulposus, which is caused by reduction of proteoglycans and is often associated with disc height decrease. Dehydration is well demonstrated by MRI because the disc becomes hypointense on T1- and T2-weighted sequences. In most cases disc dehydration is asymptomatic, but it indicates disc overload and often is followed by further degenerative abnormalities. In more advanced cases, degeneration progresses with wide destruction of the disc, extreme height reduction, and intradiscal gas formation. Gas frequently is observed on CT as an air density intradiscal area. MRI is less accurate for identifying gas, which appears as a hypointense area on all sequences.

Another common disc alteration is the intranuclear cleft, an early sign of disc degeneration caused by transverse rupture of nuclear fibers that appears as a hypointense transverse band inside the nucleus pulposus (Fig. 17A). This finding appears in all

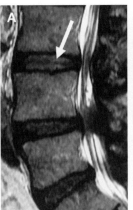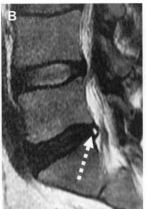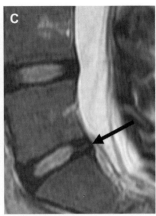

Fig. 17. Disc fissures. (*A*) On sagittal T2-weighted MRI intranuclear cleft appears as a low signal intranuclear straight line (*arrow*). (*B*) Circumferential fissure appears on Fast Spin-Echo T2-weighted sagittal image as a small round hyperintense area (*arrow*). (*C*) Radial fissure is visible on T2-weighted MRI as a straight, hyperintense area radiating from the nucleus into the annulus (*black arrow*).

discs in the adult population after 40 years, and it is considered a paraphysiologic asymptomatic change.

Degenerative changes of the annular fibers may result in two types of fissures [7]: (1) circumferential fissures and (2) radial fissures. The former type consists of rupture of collagen bridges among annular fibers with annular weakness and preserved integrity of fibers. This alteration precedes the formation of annular bulging. On sagittal T2-weighted MRI, circumferential fissure appears as a focal hyperintense area into the external aspect of the annulus (Fig. 17B). Radial fissure is a linear rupture of annular fibers extending from the nucleus pulposus. Radial fissure can progress to more severe disruption and determine disc herniation. Rupture of inner thin, annular fibers leads to protrusion and rupture of thick peripheral fibers to herniation. On MRI, radial fissure appears as a hyperintense transverse band into the annulus (Fig. 17C). Radial and circumferential fissures have been found to determine microinstability and increased mobility of the discosomatic unit [26,27].

In the literature and in clinical practice, the definition of the forms of disc degeneration is often not univocal, because different terms are used for the same entity and vice versa. Recently, an attempt to define standard and uniform terminology was made [28]. According to the new nomenclature, in the bulging disc the contour of the outer annulus extends in the axial plane beyond the edges of the disc space over more than 50% of the circumference of the disc and usually less than 3 mm beyond the edges of the vertebral body (Fig. 18A). The bulging is defined as asymmetric if it is more evident in one section of the periphery of the disc but is not so focal as to be characterized as a protrusion. Disc

herniation is defined as localized displacement of disc material beyond the normal margins of the intervertebral disc space. Disc herniation is classified as protrusion or extrusion.

> Protrusion means that the greatest distance, in any plane, between the edges of the disc material beyond the disc space is less than the distance between the edges at the base in the same plane (Fig. 18B).
> Extrusion means that any one distance between the edges of the disc material beyond the disc space is greater than the distance between the edges of the base in the same plane (Fig. 18C). When no contiguity exists with the parent disc, the extruded material may be characterized as sequester or free fragment (Fig. 18D).

Other definitions include the concept of migrated disc and contained herniation. In the migrated disc a portion of herniated disc material is displaced away from the tear in the outer annulus through which it has extruded. Contained herniation is defined as displaced disc tissue that is wholly within an outer perimeter of uninterrupted outer annulus or capsule. If the annulus is completely interrupted, the herniation can be defined as uncontained. When the herniation crosses the posterior longitudinal ligament, it can be defined as extraligamentous or transligamentous. This event is uncommon, and the fragment does not migrate for more than one level because of the strict adhesion of the Trolard's ligament to the vertebral body in the midline. Relative to the axial plane, the herniation may be (1) central, (2) right-left central, (3) right-left subarticular, (4) right-left foraminal, or (5) right-left extraforaminal.

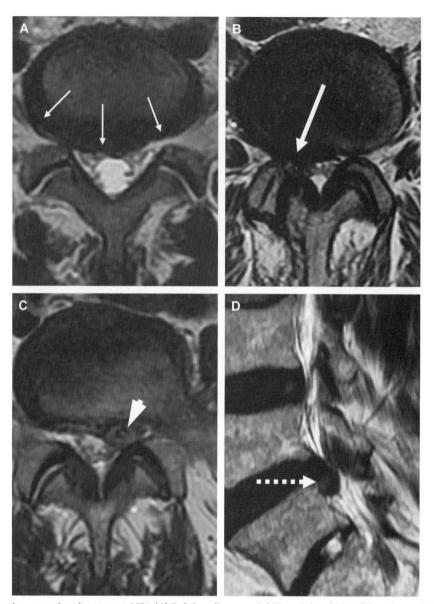

Fig. 18. Disc degenerative changes on MRI. (*A*) Bulging disc on axial T2-weighted MRI. (*B*) Right-central disc protrusion demonstrated on axial T2-weighted MRI. (*C*) Subarticular disc extrusion (note that the herniated material is hyperintense, a favorable prognostic sign) observed on T2-weighted MRI. (*D*) Sagittal T2-weighted MRI shows migrated herniation with preserved continuity with the disc.

CT is accurate for the diagnosis of disc herniation and allows the differential diagnosis between bulging and herniation, the evaluation of dimensions and location of the herniated disc, and the detection of free fragments. The disc is hypodense but the nucleus pulposus cannot be exactly identified. CT is more accurate than MRI for the identification of calcified herniations and associated bony abnormalities, such as posterior accompanying osteophytes, which can be important for therapeutic decisions [7,10].

MRI is the technique most frequently used for the evaluation of disc herniation. The examination should comprise sagittal T1- and T2-weighted sequences and axial T1- and/or T2-weighted sequences. In the cervical tract, axial GE T2-weighted sequences are useful for differentiating osteophytes and disc material. MRI is the optimal diagnostic tool, comparable in sensitivity to myelo-CT, for the diagnosis of disc herniation. The principle of disc herniation diagnosis is the same with CT and MRI. The herniation is seen as a focal contour abnormality along the posterior disc margin with a soft tissue mass displacing the epidural fat and, sometimes, the dural sac and the nerve roots. The herniation is usually contiguous with the rest of the disc, but free fragments are possible [1,7,29]. The herniation is usually isointense to the rest of the disc on T1- and T2-weighted sequences. The herniation often is slightly or strongly hyperintense on T2-weighted sequences, however [7].

After gadolinium injection, many herniations have a thin peripheral enhancing rim caused by the inflammatory reaction [30]. Contrast injection is usually not necessary, however, but in select cases it can be useful for differential diagnosis between herniation and neurinoma. Contrast agent is more widely used in postoperative examinations, because it is useful for differentiating residual or recurrent herniations from scar tissue.

MRI is sensitive to the detection of early changes of the disc anatomy. This examination sometimes leads to an overinterpretation of the findings, giving pathologic meaning to paraphysiologic features and vice versa. Patient history and symptoms must be evaluated with care. Correlation with MRI findings is important to find out the reason for symptoms and give indication of surgery or other invasive treatments.

Natural history

Disc herniations usually have a favorable outcome. Long-term follow-up studies showed that regression or reduction of symptoms occurred in 71% to 95% of patients after 1 year, and stability or worsening occurred in 5% to 29% of patients [31–33]. Follow-up of surgically and non–surgically treated patients indicate that after a 5- to 10-year period,

the success rate is similar [34–36]. Indications for surgery are actually selective because conservative treatment is usually effective.

Imaging studies with MRI follow-up 6 to 12 months after the diagnosis demonstrated that 63% of disc herniations may show a spontaneous volume reduction [31,37,38]. The causes of spontaneous reduction of herniated disc material are shrinkage caused by dehydration, fragmentation, and phagocytosis of the disc material. Shrinkage and fragmentation are related to matrix degeneration and loss of proteoglycans integrity; phagocytosis is induced by local inflammation with an immunomediated process, because nucleus pulposus is immunologically segregated [39].

MRI can be used for follow-up of nontreated disc herniations [30,40,41]. The main MRI findings useful to presume spontaneous regression of disc herniations after 6 months are [41] free fragments (100%), T2-weighted hyperintense herniation (83%), peripheral enhancement after gadolinium administration (80%), and recent clinical onset (75%). Among the types of herniations, protrusions are usually more stable than extrusions. Bulging disc history is different, because it usually does not undergo spontaneous anatomic regression and symptoms are more stable.

Finally, radiology is involved not only in the diagnostic phase of degenerative disc disease but also in the therapeutic phase [42]. Many minimally invasive interventional radiology techniques have been designed: automated discectomy [43], percutaneous laser disc decompression [44], coblation and intradiscal oxygen-ozone injection (chemiodiscolysis) (Fig. 19) [45]. All these technique offer a valid

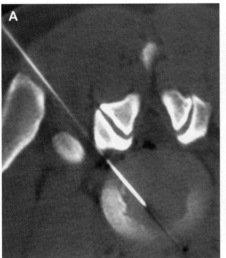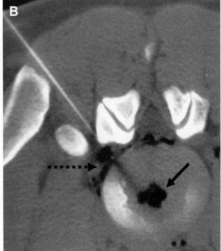

Fig. 19. Oxygen-ozone chemiodiscolysis of left L5-S1 protrusion. (*A*) CT-guided left paravertebral access to the nucleus pulposus. (*B*) Wide distribution of the hypodense gas into the nucleus (*arrow*), the perigangliar area (*dotted arrow*), and the epidural space is shown.

alternative to surgery, because at follow-up their success rate ranges from 70% to 80% [45]. Their potential complications are minimal and there is no risk of failed back surgery syndrome.

References

[1] Gallucci M, Puglielli E, Splendiani A, et al. Degenerative disorders of the spine. Eur Radiol 2005;15:591–8.

[2] Resnick D. Degenerative disease of the vertebral column. Radiology 1985;156:3–14.

[3] Rabishong P. Comprehensive approach to the discoradicular conflict. Rivista di Neuroradiologia 1997;10:515–8.

[4] Ruschalleda J, Feliciani M, Rovira A. Degenerative changes of lumbosacral spine. Rivista di Neuroradiologia 1995;8(s1):177–96.

[5] Modic MT, Masaryk TJ, Ross JS, et al. Imaging of degenerative disk disease. Radiology 1988;168: 177–86.

[6] Simonetti L, Menditto M, Sirabella G, et al. L'invecchiamento del rachide. Rivista di Neuroradiologia 1994;7(s3):53–62.

[7] Czervionke LF, Haughton VM. Degenerative disease of the spine. In: Atlas SW, editor. Magnetic resonance imaging of the brain and spine. Philadelphia: Lippincott-Raven Publisher; 2002. p. 1633–714.

[8] Deyo RA, Weinstein JN. Low back pain. N Engl J Med 2001;344:363–70.

[9] Almen A, Tingberg A, Besjakov J, et al. The use of reference image criteria in X-ray diagnostics: can application for the optimisation of lumbar spine radiographs. Eur Radiol 2004;14:1561–7.

[10] Czervionke LF. Lumbar intervertebral disc disease. Neuroimaging Clin N Am 1993;3:465–85.

[11] Cartolari R. Functional evaluation of the operated lumbar spine with axial loaded computed tomography (AL-CT). Rivista di Neuroradiologia 2002;15:393–8.

[12] Hiwatashi A, Danielson B, Moritani T, et al. Axial loading during MR imaging can influence treatment decision for symptomatic spinal stenosis. AJNR Am J Neuroradiol 2004;25:170–4.

[13] Jinkins JR, Dworkin JS, Damadian RV. Upright, weight-bearing, dynamic-kinetic MRI of the spine: initial results. Eur Radiol 2005;15: 1815–25.

[14] Jensen MC, Brant-Zawadzki MN, Obuchowski N, et al. Magnetic resonance imaging of the lumbar spine in people without back pain. N Engl J Med 1994;331:69–73.

[15] Modic MT. Degenerative disc disease and back pain. Magn Reson Imaging Clin N Am 1999;7: 481–91.

[16] Modic MT, Steinberg PM, Ross JS, et al. Degenerative disc disease: assessment of changes in vertebral body marrow with MR imaging. Radiology 1988;166:194–9.

[17] Mitra D, Cassar-Pullicino VN, McCall IW. Longitudinal study of vertebral type-1 end-plate changes on MR of the lumbar spine. Eur Radiol 2004;14:1573–81.

[18] Jinkins JR. Acquired degenerative changes of the intervertebral segments at and suprajacent to the lumbosacral junction: a radioanatomic analysis of the nondiscal structures of the spinal column and perispinal soft tissues. Eur J Radiol 2004;50: 134–58.

[19] Helbig T, Lee CK. The lumbar facet syndrome. Spine 1988;13:61–4.

[20] Murtagh R. The art and science of nerve root and facet blocks. Neuroimaging Clin N Am 2000;10: 465–77.

[21] Rossi F, Dragoni S. Lumbar spondylolysis and sports: the radiological findings and statistical considerations. Radiol Med (Torino) 1994;87: 397–400.

[22] Harvey CJ, Richenberg JL, Saifuddin A, et al. The radiological investigation of lumbar spondylolysis. Clin Radiol 1998;53:723–8.

[23] Jayakumar P, Nnadi C, Saifuddin A, et al. Dynamic degenerative lumbar spondylolisthesis: diagnosis with axial loaded magnetic resonance imaging. Spine 2006;31:E298–301.

[24] Congeni J, Mc Culloch J, Swanson K. Lumbar spondylolysis: a study of natural progression in athletes. Am J Sports Med 1997;2:248–53.

[25] Yoshida M, Shima K, Taniguchi Y. Hypertrophied ligamentum flavum in lumbar canal spinal stenosis: pathogenesis, morphologic and immunohistochemical observation. Spine 1992;17: 1353–60.

[26] Saifuddin A, McSweeney E, Lehovsky J. Development of lumbar high intensity zone on axial loaded magnetic resonance imaging. Spine 2003; 28:E449–51.

[27] Haughton VM, Rogers B, Meyerand ME, et al. Measuring the axial rotation of lumbar vertebrae in vivo with MR imaging. AJNR Am J Neuroradiol 2002;23:1110–6.

[28] Fardon DF, Milette PC. Nomenclature and classification of lumbar disc pathology: recommendations of the combined task forces of the North American Spine Society, American Society of Spine Radiology, and American Society of Neuroradiology. Spine 2001;26:E93–113.

[29] Milette PC, Fontaine S, Lepanto L, et al. Differentiating lumbar disc protrusions, disc bulges, and discs with normal contour but abnormal signal intensity: magnetic resonance imaging with discographic correlations. Spine 1999;24:44–53.

[30] Gallucci M, Bozzao A, Orlandi B, et al. Does postcontrast MR enhancement in lumbar disk herniation have prognostic value? J Comput Assist Tomogr 1995;19:34–8.

[31] Bozzao A, Gallucci M, Masciocchi C, et al. Lumbar disk herniation: MR imaging assessment of natural history in patients treated without surgery. Radiology 1992;185:35–141.

[32] Saal JA. Natural history and nonoperative treatment of lumbar disc herniation. Spine 1996;21: 2S–9S.

[33] Bush K, Cowan N, Katz DE, et al. The natural history of sciatica associated with disc pathology: a prospective study with clinical and independent radiologic follow-up. Spine 1992;17:1205–12.

[34] Komori H, Shinomiya K, Nakai O, et al. The natural history of herniated nucleus pulposus with radiculopathy. Spine 1996;21:225–9.

[35] Davis RA. A long-term outcome analysis of 984 surgically treated herniated lumbar discs. J Neurosurg 1994;80:415–21.

[36] Postacchini F. Spine update: results of surgery compared with conservative management for lumbar disc herniations. Spine 1996;21:1383–7.

[37] Gallucci M, Bozzao A, Orlandi B, et al. Follow-up of surgically treated and untreated disk pathology. Rivista di Neuroradiologia 1995;8(s1):85–96.

[38] Delauche-Cavallier MC, Budet C, Laredo JD, et al. Lumbar disc herniation: computed tomography scan changes after conservative treatment of nerve root compression. Spine 1992;17:927–33.

[39] McCarron RF, Wimpee MW, Hudkins P. The inflammatory effect of nucleus pulposus: a possible element in the pathogenesis of low back pain. Spine 1987;12:760–4.

[40] Kawaji Y, Uchiyama S, Yagi E. Three-dimensional evaluation of lumbar disc hernia and prediction of absorption by enhanced MRI. J Orthop Sci 2001;6:498–502.

[41] Splendiani A, Puglielli E, De Amicis R, et al. Spontaneous resolution of lumbar disk herniation: predictive signs for prognostic evaluation. Neuroradiology 2004;46:916–22.

[42] El-Khoury GY, Renfrew DL. Percutaneous procedures for the diagnosis and treatment of lower back pain: discography, facet-joint injection, and epidural injection. AJR Am J Roentgenol 1991;157:685–91.

[43] Bonaldi G. Automated percutaneous lumbar discectomy: technique, indications and clinical follow-up in over 1000 patients. Neuroradiology 2003;45:735–43.

[44] Choy D, Ascher P, Ranu HS, et al. Percutaneous laser disc decompression: a new therapeutic modality. Spine 1992;17:440–3.

[45] Gallucci M, Limbucci N, Zugaro L, et al. Sciatica: treatment with intradiscal and intraforaminal injections of steroid and oxygen–ozone versus steroid only. Radiology 2007;242:907–13.

NEUROIMAGING
CLINICS
OF NORTH AMERICA

Neuroimag Clin N Am 17 (2007) 105–115

Scoliosis

Johan Van Goethem, MD, PhD[a,b,*], A. Van Campenhout, MD[c],
Luc van den Hauwe, MD[a], Paul M. Parizel, MD, PhD[a]

In the frontal plane, the normal load-bearing spine is straight. Scoliosis is a structural lateral curvature of the spine with a rotatory component. A small deviation (<10°) is sometimes called spinal asymmetry, whereas "true" scoliosis has a deviation of ≥10°. This deviation is accompanied by a rotation that is maximally at the apex of the curve. In the thoracic region, this rotation creates an asymmetry of the thoracic cage that produces the typical chest wall prominence known as the Adams sign.

Imaging in scoliosis is important. Most cases of scoliosis are idiopathic, and imaging is used routinely in monitoring the changes of the deformity that take place during growth. Imaging is also crucial in determining the underlying etiology in non-idiopathic cases of scoliosis and is used in pre- and postoperative monitoring.

Generally, scoliosis is treated by orthopedic surgeons who have special training in spinal and pediatric problems. Patients who have scoliosis may present directly to the radiology department through a primary health care physician or may be referred from the pediatric, neurology, or neurosurgery departments. Many physicians look toward the radiologist as the spinal expert. Therefore, radiologists should know the basics of scoliosis, how to perform the radiologic examination, how to read these films correctly, and how to make a coherent and helpful interpretation.

Classification

Scoliosis can be classified according to etiology, curve location, age at onset, and curve type.

Etiology

Congenital scoliosis
Congenital scoliosis is the most frequent congenital spinal deformity. It is present at birth as the result of

[a] Department of Radiology, University of Antwerp, Wilrijkstraat 10, B2650 Edegem (Antwerp), Belgium
[b] Department of Radiology, AZ Nikolaas, Hospitaalstraat 8, B9100 Sint-Niklaas, Belgium
[c] Department of Orthopaedics, University Hospitals Leuven, Pellenberg, Weligerveld 1, 3212 Pellenberg, Belgium
* Corresponding author. Department of Radiology, University of Antwerp, Wilrijkstraat 10, B2650 Edegem (Antwerp), Belgium.
E-mail address: johan.vangoethem@ua.ac.be (J. Van Goethem).

doi:10.1016/j.nic.2006.12.001

embryologic or intrauterine maldevelopment of vertebral elements. The term "congenital" is slightly misleading because it implies that the curvature is apparent at birth, but this is not necessarily so. The vertebral anomalies are present at birth, and the clinical deformity develops with spinal growth and may not become apparent until later childhood [1]. These may be caused by failure of formation or failure of segmentation. They are commonly associated with cardiac or urologic abnormalities that develop during the same period (before 48 days of gestation) (Fig. 1) [2]. Vertebral maldevelopment can be classified as defects of segmentation or defects of formation. Curve progression is strongly related to the type of vertebral abnormality with the poorest prognosis for unilateral unsegmented bars with contralateral hemivertebrae (up to 10°/yr progression), a less severe progression in

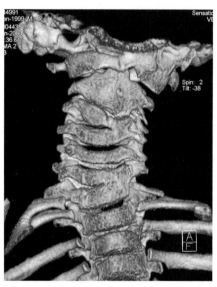

Fig. 1. A 5-year-old boy who has Klippel-Feil syndrome type II. Klippel-Feil syndrome occurs in a heterogeneous group of patients unified only by the presence of a congenital defect in the formation or segmentation of the cervical spine [2]. Numerous associated abnormalities of other organ systems may be present. As a consequence of these fusion and segmentation anomalies, this patient has a congenital cervical and thoracic scoliosis. Klippel-Feil type I shows massive fusion of cervical and upper thoracic vertebrae. Type II shows fusion of a limited number of vertebrae and hemivertebrae. Occipitoatlantal fusion and other lower thoracic anomalies are present. Type III shows cervical fusions and lower thoracic or lumbar fusions. C2-C3 fusion, also present in this case, is the most common form of congenital fused cervical vertebrae and is probably dominant with variable expression. This patient also shows hemivertebrae and unilateral fused vertebrae.

cases of hemivertebrae or double hemivertebrae (1–2.5° and 2–5°/yr, respectively), and a least severe progression in patients who have block and wedge vertebrae (<1°/yr progression) (Fig. 2). The most common anomaly is hemivertebrae, which is seen in about 40% of cases.

Idiopathic scoliosis

Most frequently, scoliosis is idiopathic (80% of cases). Substantial research efforts have identified several factors contributing to the development of idiopathic scoliosis.

Genetic factors are a potential etiologic component in the development of scoliosis. There is evidence for several different modes of inheritance, including multifactorial, autosomal dominant, and X-linked dominant, with variable phenotypic expression. Several candidate regions have been identified, including on chromosomes 6p, distal 10q, 17p11, 18q, and 19p13 [3]. Family members of affected individuals have an increased incidence of scoliosis. Studies in families with twins have identified 73% to 92% concordance in monozygotic twins and only 36% to 63% concordance in dizygotic twins. The prevalence of scoliosis increases seven times in individuals who have affected siblings and three times in those who have affected parents.

Idiopathic scoliosis is apparently a result of inadequate control of spinal growth. The deformity progresses most rapidly during adolescent growth, and there is evidence that adolescents who have idiopathic scoliosis have an earlier growth spurt [4], are taller and thinner, and have an increased level of growth hormone.

Vertebral growth anomalies may be related to adolescent idiopathic scoliosis. Differential growth rates between left and right sides of the spine may lead to asymmetry that could be accentuated by the Heuter-Volkmann effect (suppression of growth on the concave side of the curve). When anterior spinal growth outpaces posterior growth in an adolescent patient, hypokyphosis is produced, with subsequent buckling of the vertebral column. Scoliotic spines in girls between 12 and 14 years of age have longer thoracic vertebral bodies, shorter pedicles, and a larger interpedicular distance compared with the spines of normal, aged-matched girls [5]. The differential growth between the anterior and posterior elements is not only significantly different in scoliosis versus normal spines but is also correlated to the severity of scoliosis. This overgrowth in length mainly occurs by enchondral ossification, whereas circumferential growth is slower and happens by membranous ossification.

A **B**

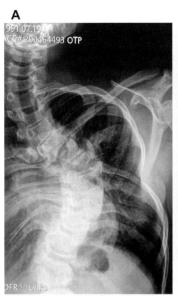

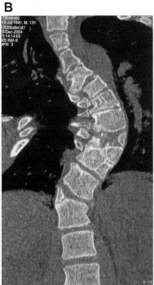

Fig. 2. Postero-anterior plain film (*A*) and multiplanar reconstruction 3-D reformation of a multi-row detector CT in a patient who has congenital thoracic scoliosis with wedge vertebrae and hemivertebrae (*B*). Curve progression is strongly related to the type of vertebral abnormality, with the poorest prognosis for unilateral unsegmented bars with contralateral hemivertebrae (up to 10°/yr progression), a less severe progression in cases of hemivertebrae or double hemivertebrae (1–2.5°/yr and 25°/yr, respectively), as in this case, and a least severe progression in patients who have block and wedge vertebrae (<1°/yr progression). Associated rib anomalies are seen frequently.

Scoliosis in generalized diseases and syndromes

Neural axis abnormalities have a prevalence between 19.5% and 26% among infantile and juvenile scoliosis cases [6]. Several factors have been identified that correlate with a higher incidence in scoliosis, such as equilibrium and vestibular dysfunction, melatonin deficiency, syringomyelia (Fig. 3), Chiari malformation, and spinal tumors. Neuromuscular disorders (eg, cerebral palsy and muscular dystrophy) and some generalized diseases and syndromes (eg, Marfan, neurofibromatosis, rheumatoid disease, or bone dysplasia) are associated with scoliosis. Scoliosis is seen in 8.7% of patients who have Down syndrome [7].

Traumatic scoliosis

Traumatic scoliosis can be caused by bony lesions (eg, fractures and dislocations) or by soft tissue lesions (eg, burns and postempyema).

Degenerative scoliosis

Degenerative lumbar scoliosis is a lateral deviation of the spine that typically develops after 50 years of age [8]. This is type 1 adult scoliosis, which is primarily degenerative. It is caused most frequently

A **B**

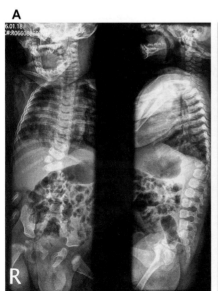

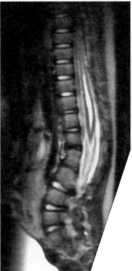

Fig. 3. Clinically suspected infantile scoliosis is confirmed by plain film (*A*). All cases of infantile and juvenile idiopathic scoliosis r͏͏ ͏ther work-up with MR ͏ ͏ ͏they are com- ͏variety

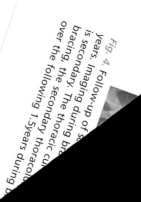

Fig. 4. Follow-up of s͏ years. Imaging during ͏ is secondary, the ͏ bracing. The thoracic ͏ over the following 1.5 years during ͏

by a disc or facet joint arthritis, affecting those structures asymmetrically. Type 2 adult scoliosis is the progression of adolescent scoliosis in adulthood. Type 3 adult scoliosis is a secondary scoliosis mostly caused by osteoporosis [9]. Although the clinical presentation may vary, degenerative scoliosis is usually associated with loss of lordosis, axial rotation, lateral listhesis, and spondylolisthesis. It is associated with degenerative disk and facet disease and hypertrophy of the ligamenta flava, typically leading to neurogenic claudication and back pain. Rarely, sagittal or coronal imbalance may develop.

Curve location

Curve location is defined by its center, known as the apex, which is the most lateral disc or vertebra of the curve. Usually the apical vertebra is also the most horizontal. Scoliosis can be classified as cervical (apex between C2 and C6), cervicothoracic (C7–T1), thoracic (T2–T11), thoracolumbar (T12–L1), lumbar (L2–L4), or lumbosacral (L5 and below).

Age at onset

Age at onset or diagnosis is used to classify scoliosis as the following types: type 1, infantile (0–3 years); type 2, juvenile (4–10 years, mean age of diagnosis of juvenile scoliosis is around 8 years); type 3, adolescent (11–17 years); and type 4, adult (≥18 years).

Curve types

Primary curves are the first to develop. Secondary curves develop as a means to balance the head and trunk over the pelvis, not only in the frontal but also in the sagittal plane. At the time of diagnosis, it is not always possible to differentiate primary curves from secondary curves (Fig. 4). Structural curves (as opposed to nonstructural curves) cannot be corrected with side-bending or traction. Nonstructural curves can be secondary curves or functional curves (postural, secondary to short leg, muscle spasm).

Several classifications according to different curve patterns have been proposed as a preoperative assessment. The use of these classification schemes allows scoliosis practitioners to compare various treatments of similar curve patterns and to recommend selective fusions of the spine when appropriate. The most widely used classification, developed by Moe and reported by King and colleagues [10] (the King-Moe Classification), was designed primarily to help the clinician to decide when to instrument the thoracic curve alone and when to instrument the thoracic and lumbar curves. This classification is not comprehensive, and a more complete and reliable classification was proposed by Lenke and colleagues [11]. The Lenke Classification considers three components: curve type (types 1–6), a lumbar spine modifier (A, B, or C), and a sagittal thoracic modifier (−, N, or +). The six curve types have specific characteristics on frontal

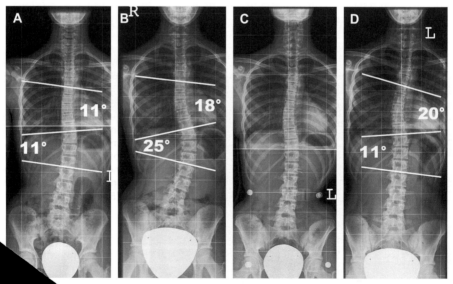

...coliosis in an adolescent girl. (*A*) 13 years. (*B*) 14 years. (*C*) 14.5 years with brace. (*D*) 15.5 ...acing confirms that the thoracic curve is structural and that the thoracolumbar curve ...rve progresses 7° between ages 13 and 14, after which bracing is started. During ...mbar curve can be partially corrected. The thoracic curve only progresses 2° ...racing.

and sagittal radiographs that differentiate structural and nonstructural curves in the proximal thoracic (PT), main thoracic (MT), and thoracolumbar/lumbar regions (TL/L). The major curve is the one with the largest Cobb measurement and is included in fusion surgery for idiopathic adolescent scoliosis. The minor curves are all other nonmajor curves. One of the main debates in scoliosis surgery is whether to include those minor curves in the fusion. Thus, six curve types are distinguished in this system based on whether the PT, MT, and TL/L regions are major, minor structural, or nonstructural, including type 1, MT; type 2, double thoracic; type 3, double major; type 4, triple major; Type 5, TL/L; Type 6, TL/L-MT [12]. Many other classification types exist, such as the Scoliosis Research Society Classification for Adult Spinal Deformity, but these usually differ mainly on surgical interpretation points.

Prevalence

The prevalence of scoliosis ($\geq 10°$) in the childhood and adolescent population is between 0.5% and 3.0%. Adolescent idiopathic scoliosis is present in 2% to 4% of children between 10 and 16 years of age. Larger curves (>30°) are reported between 0.04% and 0.29%. In childhood scoliosis, 0.5% is reported in the infantile group, 10% in the juvenile group, and the remainder in the adolescent group.

Clinical features

There is no difference in the prevalence of back pain or mortality between patients who have untreated adolescent idiopathic scoliosis and the general population. Patients who have mild idiopathic scoliosis (<25°) usually have little or no discomfort. Cardiopulmonary complications are almost exclusively seen in early-onset scoliosis (<5 years of age). Patients presenting with severe pain, neurologic symptoms, or rapidly progressing scoliosis require thorough further examination. In adults, degenerative scoliosis may contribute significantly to facet joint degeneration and spinal and foraminal stenosis with subsequent clinical symptomatology.

Infantile idiopathic scoliosis presents as a left thoracic curve in 90% of cases. The male/female ratio is 3:2. In juvenile idiopathic scoliosis, the male/female ratio is 1:2 to 1:4; boys are more affected between 3 and 6 years of age (1:1), and girls are more affected between 6 and 10 years of age (1:8). The number of right and left curves is equal in the younger group (<6 years at presentation), and right curves predominate in the older group (80%).

In North America and Europe, a screening examination in school often leads to a first referral for scoliosis. The goal of school screening programs is to detect childhood scoliosis at a stage where surgical correction can be avoided.

Clinical tests are available to assess scoliosis. The forward-bend test or Adams test is probably the best known. In this test, the patient bends forward with the knees straight and the palms together. During this test, the thoracic and lumbar regions should stay symmetric. An asymmetric rotational hump of 5° to 7° is associated with a scoliosis of 15° to 20°. A referral and imaging is recommended when the angle of trunk rotation is greater than 7°. This is a sensitive, although not a specific, test (2–3% referral).

Natural history

Congenital scoliosis

Congenital scoliosis shows progression in 75% of cases. The poorest prognosis is for thoracic curves and for multiple hemivertebrae and a convex unilateral bar (failure of segmentation) opposite the hemivertebrae. Block and wedge vertebrae show progression <1°/yr, hemivertebrae show a mean progression of 1° to 2.5°/yr, double hemivertebrae increase at a double rate, and unilateral unsegmented bars with contralateral vertebrae may progress up to 10°/yr. The management of congenital scoliosis requires frequent clinical and radiographic follow-up to detect progression. Curve progression or severe vertebral anomalies known to cause curve progression require prompt treatment to prevent deformity and morbidity, such as thoracic insufficiency syndrome [13].

Infantile idiopathic scoliosis

The vast majority of these curves are self-limiting. The few that progress (usually double structural curves) can be difficult to manage. In cases where the rib vertebral angle difference is larger than 20°, progression is likely. The rib vertebral angle difference is defined as the difference in angulation of the left and right ribs on the apical vertebra as measured on an anteroposterior (AP) radiograph.

Juvenile idiopathic scoliosis

Juvenile idiopathic scoliosis is often progressive (70%). The potential for trunk deformity with cardiac and pulmonary compromise exists especially in scoliosis with onset before 5 years of age. Curves of greater than 30° are almost always progressive, at a rate of 1° to 3°/yr before 10 years of age and at a rate of 4.5° to 11°/yr after 10 years of age. If the scoliosis is in the thoracic region, surgery is required in more than 95% of these cases.

Adolescent idiopathic scoliosis

Roughly 2% of adolescents have a scoliosis (>10°), but only 5% of these have a progression of the curve to greater than 30° (Fig. 4). The progression of scoliosis is dependent on the growth velocity and the magnitude of the curve at the first visit. Progression is most notable with a growth velocity of greater than 2 cm/yr, between 9 and 13 years of age, at bone ages between 9 and 14 years, at Risser signs 0 to 1, and between 0.5 and 2 years before menarche [14].

The key risk factors for curve progression are the remaining spinal growth (skeletal immaturity) combined with the curve magnitude at a given time and, to a lesser degree, female gender [15]. Skeletal immaturity or remaining skeletal growth is determined by age, menarchal status, and Risser sign (radiologic) or Tanner staging (clinical). The main progression occurs at the time of most rapid skeletal growth. This occurs at 11 to 13 years of age for girls and at 13 to 15 years of age for boys. Determining the peak height velocity (PHV) timing by accurate serial heights measurements is difficult. Usually, patients present without accurate prior height measurements. In these cases, other markers have to be used. The Risser stage is still 0 at the time of PHV, and this phase of accelerated skeletal growth is split into halves by the closure of the triradiate cartilage [16]. Other markers can be used, including digital uncapped phalangeal epiphyses, which are indicative of pre-PHV, and fused epiphyses, which are indicative of post-PHV. Capped but nonfused epiphyses are indeterminant. Tanner stage 1 for breast strongly indicates pre-PHV. Stage 3 for breast and pubic hair occurs at or after the PHV, and stage 4 occurrs after PHV [17]. In the decelerating growth phase, a Risser less than 1 is associated with progression in 60% to 70% of patients, whereas Risser 3 has a risk for progression in less than 10%. Curve pattern has also been identified as an important variable for predicting the probability of progression. Primary thoracic curve scoliosis, especially King types II, III, and V, progress more than primary lumbar curve scoliosis.

Adult idiopathic scoliosis

Curves of less than 30° usually show no progression. Curves measuring 30° to 50° at skeletal maturity progress at an average of 10° to 15° during a normal lifetime. Curves between 50° and 75° show a continuing rate of nearly 1°/yr. In untreated patients, an increased mortality rate due to cardiopulmonary disorders is seen most frequently in scoliosis of greater than 90°.

Imaging in scoliosis

Plain film imaging technique

The ideal imaging modality for screening in scoliosis is the upright posteroanterior radiograph of the entire spine (Fig. 4). The head and pelvis should be on the same film. The patient must be standing, but in young patients or patients who have severe neuromuscular disorders, a sitting or supine radiograph may be the only possibility. In general, no attempt should be made to equalize differences in leg length. A lateral film is not required as a part of the screening examination.

Radiographic techniques should be used to minimize radiation of sensitive organs (eg, breast, thyroid, ovaries, bone marrow, and lens). It is imperative that radiation-lowering techniques are used judiciously to minimize the radiation burden. In a recent study of 5,466 women who received an average of 24.7 radiographs with a mean estimated cumulative radiation dose to the breast of 10.8 cGy (range, 0–170 cGy), the risk of breast cancer was found to be 70% higher than in women in the general population [18]. There were 77 breast cancer deaths among these patients, compared with 46 expected deaths based on United States mortality rates. Risk increased significantly with increasing number of radiograph exposures and with cumulative radiation dose. A posterior-to-anterior technique reduces radiation to the breast 3 to 7 fold compared with an anterior-to-posterior technique. If breast shielding is used, one should take care that automatic exposure systems do not increase the radiation dose accordingly. A further decrease in radiation dose can be accomplished using the air-gap technique. This technique was first described in 1934 by Lindblom [19]. In clinical practice, it was soon superseded by the use of anti-scatter grids. Air gaps are still used in lung examinations and compare favorably with the use of grids in pediatric radiology. The introduction of digital radiography is likely to create a new interest in the air-gap technique [20]. With air-gap and computed radiology techniques, the mean effective dose can be reduced by a factor of 10 [21].

When surgical treatment is considered, lateral bend radiographs and a lateral film should be acquired. Bend films aid in deciding what levels should be included in the instrumentation (Fig. 5). Lateral bending is usually performed as a standing postero-anterior film, but in some institutions supine AP films are used. The Stagnara oblique view is taken perpendicularly to the rib prominence and shows a more accurate picture of large curves with a true magnitude of the scoliosis.

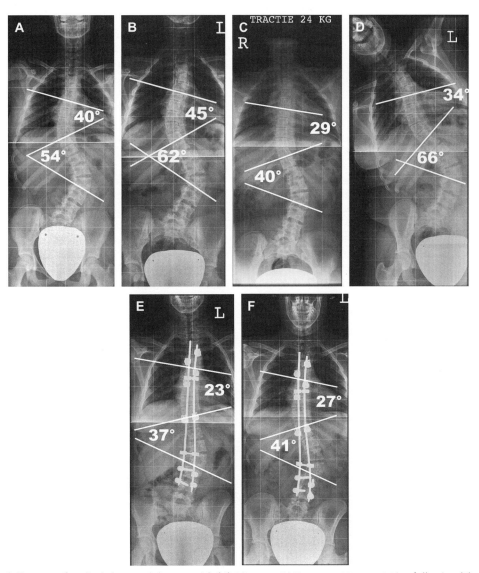

Fig. 5. Follow-up of scoliosis in an adolescent girl. (*A*) 14 years. 14.5-years postero-anterior full spine (*B*) under traction (*C*) and with lateral bending (*D*). Postoperative postero-anterior full spine at 15 years (*E*) and 16 years (*F*). Curve progression of 5° thoracic and 8° lumbar in 6 months warranted surgical stabilization. Before surgery traction and lateral bend, films are used to determine which curves are structural (both were structural in this case) and the extent of the surgical fixation. Surgery reduced the curves with 22° and 25°, respectively. Both curves progress 4° in the year after surgery.

Several studies have used three-dimensional (3-D) techniques to evaluate idiopathic scoliosis. These have showed that although the deformity of the spine is 3-D, the regional deformity is almost always two dimensional, but in a plane different from the standard frontal or sagittal views.

Sagittal balance is an important concept in normal spinal stability. Thoracic kyphosis and lumbosacral lordosis help to maintain a normal posture with minimum energy expenditure and absorb the loads applied to the spinal column. Many studies have shown the negative effects of a reduced lumbar lordosis with fixed sagittal imbalance after spinal instrumentation [22].

Imaging interval

Follow-up is necessary in patients who have severe curves that are at risk for significant curve progression or require some form of treatment. Idiopathic curves should be monitored every 4 to 12 months, depending on the age and growth rate of the patient (see Fig. 4). After skeletal maturity, only curves greater than 30° should be monitored for progression and usually only every 5 years.

Measurements

Curve measurement is usually performed by the Cobb method (Fig. 6). The caudal and cranial end vertebrae of a scoliosis are the most tilted in a frontal plane. A line parallel to the superior endplate of the cranial end vertebra and a line parallel to the inferior endplate of the caudal end vertebra are drawn first (on film or digitally on a diagnostic workstation). Then perpendiculars to these lines are drawn, and the angle is measured where these lines cross. A Cobb angle is measured for each curve that is present. When comparing different radiographs, the endvertebrae usually remain the same, although corrections can be needed over time. There is a wide inter- and intraobserver variation with this technique, usually in the order of 5°.

Cobb angle measurements are done on anteroposterior radiographs. Because of the associated vertebral rotation, these are not true AP views of the rotated spinal segment. Cobb angle measurements can increase by more than 20% when measured on these true AP views [23]. Therefore, in the follow-up of scoliosis, consistent patient positioning is of utmost importance.

For surgeons, it is important to recognize the important decrease of curves in the frontal and sagittal plane due to prone positioning, anesthesia, and exposure during surgery. When patients resume their standing position, a "spring-back" effect is noted in the sagittal plane with loss of correction [24].

The Ferguson Method is used much less frequently than the Cobb angle measurement. The Ferguson Method measures the angle between lines drawn from the centers of the end vertebrae to the center of the apical vertebra/disc.

As a result of the increased appreciation of the 3-D nature of scoliosis and modern spinal instrumentation's improved corrective capabilities, there has been renewed interest in the correction and measurement of vertebral rotation [25]. Vertebral rotation is maximal at the apex of the curve and can be quantified by different methods, all of which are inaccurate. CT is limited in its clinical utility owing to cost, radiation exposure, and the effects of postural changes on scoliosis curves and consequently vertebral rotation. Therefore, and because of their simplicity, the Perdriolle [26] and Nash-Moe [27] techniques remain the standard measurements for providing a reasonable estimate of pre- and postoperative vertebral rotation.

On lateral films, sagittal balance can be assessed. Normal sagittal balance is the alignment of C7 to

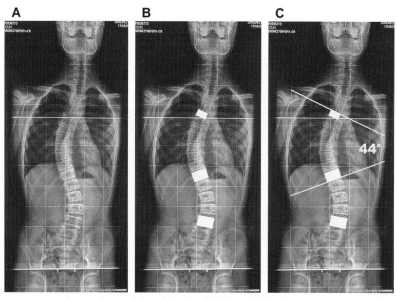

A **B** **C**

44°

Fig. 6. Curve measurement is usually performed by the Cobb method. These measurements are repeated for each curve present, in this case thoracic (apex T9) and lumbar (apex L3) (*A*). The caudal and cranial end vertebrae of each scoliosis are the most tilted in a frontal plane (T5 and T12 for the thoracic curve) (*B*). A line parallel to the superior endplate of the cranial end vertebra and a line parallel to the inferior endplate of the caudal end vertebra are drawn first (*C*). The Cobb angle is measured for each curve that is present (44° for the thoracic curve in this case). When comparing different radiographs, the endvertebrae usually remain the same (see Figs. 4 and 5), although corrections can be needed over time.

the posterior superior aspect of the sacrum. The sagittal plumb line, as drawn from center of C7, should be ±2 cm from the sacral promontory. Thoracic kyphosis depends mostly on the spinal deformity, whereas lumbar lordosis is influenced mainly by the pelvic configuration. The scoliotic curve type is not associated with a specific pattern of sagittal pelvic morphology and balance [28]. Positive sagittal balance (ie, an anterior deviation of the C7 plumb line) is more significantly associated with pain and disability than curve magnitude, curve location, or coronal imbalance [29].

Skeletal maturity is usually assessed using the Risser sign. The lateral to medial ossification of the iliac crest occurs in a predictable fashion over an 18- to 24-month period. Risser 0 is the absence of ossification, Risser stages 1 to 4 correspond to partial ossification, and Risser 5 indicates the fusion of the fully ossified apophysis to the ilium. Another useful landmark is the status of the triradiate cartilage of the acetabulum. This usually closes before Risser 0, at the stage of maximal spinal growth.

Specialized imaging

CT, especially multi-row detector CT, is the best method for visualization of complex scoliotic deformities. In general, it is used in cases of computer-assisted surgery because the placement of pedicles screws on the concavity in the apical region of thoracic curves can be critical because of small endosteal pedicle width [30]. CT is also useful to define abnormalities and to pick up previously unrecognized anomalies in patients who have congenital scoliosis [31]. The excision of hemivertebra is a technically challenging procedure and can be performed as an anterior–posterior procedure or an isolated posterior procedure, and the use of CT is helpful in the operative planning of these patients [32]. Most surgeons prefer multi-row detector CT with 3-D reconstructions over planar CT in the preoperative depiction of congenital scoliosis [33]. MR imaging is required in infantile and juvenile idiopathic scoliosis (see Fig. 3), congenital bony anomalies, and scoliosis associated with specific neurologic or cutaneous abnormalities.

The prevalence of neural axis abnormalities in infantile and juvenile idiopathic scoliosis with a curve of more than 20° is approximately 20% [34]. These include Chiari malformations, syringomyelia, and, less frequently, spinal or brain tumors. In adolescent idiopathic scoliosis, MR imaging should be considered in cases where any of these red flags is present [35] (eg, severe pain, a left thoracic curve, or an abnormal neurologic examination).

A more recent study indicates that pain as a sole indicator is not reliable for detecting pathology [36]. An atypical curve pattern most frequently is the only indicator of abnormal MR imaging findings. This includes left thoracic curve, short-segment scoliosis (4–6 levels), decreased vertebral rotation, absence of thoracic apical segment lordosis, and rapid progression. Other curve patterns are associated with an increased incidence of neural axis abnormalities, including left thoracic, double thoracic, triple thoracic, and a long right thoracic curve with end vertebra caudal to T12, and with a high or low apex or end vertebra, especially in male patients and in patients who have a normal to hyperkyphotic thoracic spine [37]. Patients who have severe curves despite skeletal immaturity and an abnormal neurologic examination have a significant probability of neurogenic lesions [38]. In patients who have juvenile idiopathic scoliosis and back pain, preoperative MR imaging should be performed to eliminate the risk of postoperative neurologic deficits, except in patients who have Lenke type 1 idiopathic scoliosis if intraoperative neural monitoring is to be performed.

Spinal cord abnormalities are seen in 3% of patients who have adolescent idiopathic scoliosis and mainly include syringomyelia and less frequently Chiari malformations [39]. Whether preoperative MR imaging in all patients who have adolescent idiopathic scoliosis is routinely indicated remains controversial [40]. The role of specialized imaging in extremely severe scoliosis remains unclear. MR screening of all patients who have scoliosis is not indicated.

Treatment

Non-operative treatment (braces)

In most cases, the aim of orthotic treatment (braces) is to avoid spinal surgery. In growing children, a spinal orthosis (brace) is indicated when a curve progresses to 25° to 30° (see Fig. 4). Lesser curves with an annual growth of more than 5° are an indication for bracing. Braces are used only in patients who have substantial remaining spinal growth (Risser 3 or less). The upper limit of curves manageable with braces is 45°. Even in the most cooperative patients, the final result of brace treatment is the maintenance of the curve degree at the level of the start of bracing. Braces should be used 23 h/d, usually for several years, until the curve is stabilized. Generally, the brace should be worn at night until skeletal maturity is reached (Risser 5 or no spinal growth for 18 months). Curve progression can be limited to less than 5° in 75% of patients, compared with 35% in a comparable nontreated group.

Surgical treatment

In general, curves greater than 45° in patients who have remaining spinal growth should be corrected surgically (see Fig. 5). Curves greater than 30° at the onset of the pubertal growth spurt increase rapidly and present a 100% prognosis for surgery. Even curves between 20° and 30° have a high progression risk and need careful follow-up. Timing of spinal surgery is of utmost importance and depends on expected curve progression. In congenital scoliosis, the curves tend to be short with little flexibility and do not show substantial response to brace treatment. Progressive congenital scoliosis is therefore generally treated with surgery. The operative treatment of adult lumbar degenerative scoliosis is a challenge, and major complication rates range from 56% to 75% [41]. Corrective instrumentation (rods) in combination with arthrodesis (strength) is the best method for achieving long-term results.

The typical posterior spinal approach uses the Harrington instrumentation. It consists of a distraction rod with hooks at either end and a threaded compression rod attached to the transverse processes on the convex side of the curve. This original concept corrected scoliosis at the cost of a decreased thoracic kyphosis. This system was subsequently modified with different systems.

The Cotrel-Dubousset system is more recent (1980s) and uses a multihook concept that allows distraction and compression on the same rod. Many of these systems can be attached with hooks, wires, or pedicle screws.

Anterior spinal instrumentation is a newer technique with several systems on the market. Initially, it was primarily used for the correction of lumbar or thoracolumbar scoliosis, but it is now also used in the thoracic region. It can also be helpful in a combination anterior and posterior approach, especially for curves larger than 75°, and in younger patients.

The correct surgical technique depends on the curve pattern. For example, in the idiopathic right thoracic curve pattern (Lenke type 1), posterior spinal instrumentation and fusion of the thoracic curve are common. The segment to be fused should be as short as possible but long enough to minimize residual imbalance or progression. The lowest hook is attached above the level where the central vertical sacral line bisects the spine. Shorter fusions are possible with anterior instrumentation, including all vertebrae in the measured Cobb angle. In a double thoracic curve (Lenke type 2), instrumentation is often extended up to T1 or T2. Different schemes exist for other patterns.

Although instrumentation generally achieves good to excellent improvement of the Cobb angle, there are conflicting reports on the long-term functional results. Complications range from blood loss over hardware failures to neurologic injury. Urinary tract infections are the most common medical complication associated with adult spinal deformity surgery. Pulmonary complications, including pneumonia and pulmonary embolism, are among the most frequently seen life-threatening complications with deformity procedures [42].

References

[1] McMaster M. Spinal growth and congenital deformity of the spine. Spine 2006;31(20):2284–7.

[2] Tracy MR, Dormans JP, Kusumi K. Klippel-Feil syndrome: clinical features and current understanding of etiology. Clin Orthop Relat Res 2004;424:183–90.

[3] Alden KJ, Marosy B, Nzegwu N, et al. Idiopathic scoliosis: identification of candidate regions on chromosome 19p13. Spine 2006;31(16):1815–9.

[4] Stokes IA, Windisch L. Vertebral height growth predominates over intervertebral disc height growth in adolescents with scoliosis. Spine 2006;31(14):1600–4.

[5] Guo X, Chau WW, Chan YL, et al. Relative anterior spinal overgrowth in adolescent idiopathic scoliosis: Results of disproportionate endochondral-membranous bone growth. J Bone Joint Surg Br 2003;85(7):1026–31.

[6] Benli IT, Uzumcugil O, Aydin E, et al. Magnetic resonance imaging abnormalities of neural axis in Lenke type 1 idiopathic scoliosis. Spine 2006; 31(16):1828–33.

[7] Milbrandt TA, Johnston CE II. Down syndrome and scoliosis: a review of a 50-year experience at one institution. Spine 2005;30(18):2051–5.

[8] Tribus CB. Degenerative lumbar scoliosis: evaluation and management. J Am Acad Orthop Surg 2003;11(3):174–83.

[9] Aebi M. The adult scoliosis. Eur Spine J 2005; 14(10):925–48.

[10] King HA, Moe JH, Bradford DS, et al. The selection of fusion levels in thoracic idiopathic scoliosis. J Bone Joint Surg Am 1983;65(9):1302–13.

[11] Lenke L, Betz R, Harms J, et al. Adolescent idiopathic scoliosis: a new classification to determine extent of spinal arthrodesis. J Bone Joint Surg Am 2001;83A:1169–81.

[12] Lenke LG, Edwards CC II, Bridwell KH. The Lenke classification of adolescent idiopathic scoliosis: how it organizes curve patterns as a template to perform selective fusions of the spine. Spine 2003;28(20):S199–207.

[13] Kose N, Campbell RM. Congenital scoliosis. Med Sci Monit 2004;10(5):104–10.

[14] Ylikoski M. Growth and progression of adolescent idiopathic scoliosis in girls. J Pediatr Orthop B 2005;14(5):320–4.

[15] Lonstein JE, Carlosn JM. The prediction of curve progression in untreated idiopathic scoliosis during growth. J Bone Joint Surg 1984;66: 1061–71.

[16] Charles YP, Daures JP, de Rosa V, et al. Progression risk of idiopathic juvenile scoliosis during pubertal growth. Spine 2006;31(17):1933–42.

[17] Sanders J, Browne R, Cooney T, et al. Correlates of the peak height velocity in girls with idiopathic scoliosis. Spine 2006;31(20):2289–95.

[18] Morin Doody M, Lonstein JE, Stovall M, et al. Breast cancer mortality after diagnostic radiography: findings from the U.S. Scoliosis Cohort Study. Spine 2002;25(16):2052–63.

[19] Lindblom K. Secondary screening by means of filtering. Acta Radiol 1934;15:620–7.

[20] Persliden J, Carlsson GA. Scatter rejection by air gaps in diagnostic radiology: Calculations using a Monte Carlo collision density method and consideration of molecular interference in coherent scattering. Phys Med Biol 1997;42:155–75.

[21] Hansen J, Jurik AG, Fiirgaard B, et al. Optimisation of scoliosis examinations in children. Pediatr Radiol 2003;33:752–65.

[22] Kim Y, Bridwell K, Lenke L, et al. An analysis of sagittal spinal alignment following long adult lumbar instrumentation and fusion to L5 or S1: can we predict ideal lumbar lordosis? Spine 2006;31(20):2343–52.

[23] Gocen S, Havitcioglu H. Effect of rotation on frontal plane deformity in idiopathic scoliosis. Orthopedics 2001;24(3):265–8.

[24] Delorme S, Labelle H, Poitras B, et al. Pre-, intra-, and postoperative three-dimensional evaluation of adolescent idiopathic scoliosis. J Spinal Disord 2000;13(2):93–101.

[25] Kuklo TR, Potter BK, Lenke LG. Vertebral rotation and thoracic torsion in adolescent idiopathic scoliosis: what is the best radiographic correlate? J Spinal Disord Tech 2005;18(2):139–47.

[26] Perdriolle R. La scoliose. Maloine, SA; Paris: 1979.

[27] Nash C, Moe J. A study of vertebral rotation. J Bone Joint Surg 1969;51:223–9.

[28] Mac-Thiong JM, Labelle H, Charlebois M, et al. Sagittal plane analysis of the spine and pelvis in adolescent idiopathic scoliosis according to the coronal curve type. Spine 2003;28(13):1404–9.

[29] Glassman SD, Bridwell K, Dimar JR. The impact of positive sagittal balance in adult spinal deformity. Spine 2005;30(18):2024–9.

[30] Liljenqvist UR, Link TM, Halm HF. Morphometric analysis of thoracic and lumbar vertebrae in idiopathic scoliosis. Spine 2000;25(10):1247–53.

[31] Newton PO, Hahn GW, Fricka KB, et al. Utility of three-dimensional and multiplanar reformatted computed tomography for evaluation of pediatric congenital spine abnormalities. Spine 2002;27(8):844–50.

[32] Hedequist DJ, Emans JB. The correlation of preoperative three-dimensional computed tomography reconstructions with operative findings in congenital scoliosis. Spine 2003;28(22):2531–4.

[33] Bush CH, Kalen V. Three-dimensional computed tomography in the assessment of congenital scoliosis. Skeletal Radiol 1999;28(11):632–7.

[34] Dobbs MB, Lenke LG, Szymanski DA, et al. Prevalence of neural axis abnormalities in patients with infantile idiopathic scoliosis. J Bone Joint Surg Am 2002;84(12):2230–4.

[35] Reamy BV, Slakey JB. Adolescent idiopathic scoliosis: review and current concepts. Am Fam Physician 2001;64(1):111–6.

[36] Davids JR, Chamberlin E, Blackhurst DW. Indications for magnetic resonance imaging in presumed adolescent idiopathic scoliosis. J Bone Joint Surg Am 2004;86-A(10):2187–95.

[37] Spiegel DA, Flynn JM, Stasikelis PJ, et al. Scoliotic curve patterns in patients with Chiari I malformation and/or syringomyelia. Spine 2003;28(18):2139–46.

[38] Morcuende JA, Dolan LA, Vazquez JD, et al. A prognostic model for the presence of neurogenic lesions in atypical idiopathic scoliosis. Spine 2004;29(1):51–8.

[39] Hausmann ON, Boni T, Pfirrmann CW, et al. Preoperative radiological and electrophysiological evaluation in 100 adolescent idiopathic scoliosis patients. Eur Spine J 2003;2(5):501–6.

[40] Do T, Fras C, Burke S, et al. Clinical value of routine preoperative magnetic resonance imaging in adolescent idiopathic scoliosis: A prospective study of three hundred and twenty-seven patients. J Bone Joint Surg Am 2001;83-A(4):577–9.

[41] Akbarnia BA, Ogilvie JW, Hammerberg KW. Debate: degenerative scoliosis: to operate or not to operate. Spine 2006;31(19):S195–201.

[42] Baron EM, Albert TJ. Medical complications of surgical treatment of adult spinal deformity and how to avoid them. Spine 2006;31(19):S106–18.

ELSEVIER
SAUNDERS

NEUROIMAGING
CLINICS
OF NORTH AMERICA

Neuroimag Clin N Am 17 (2007) 117–136

Cutting-Edge Imaging of the Spine

A. Talia Vertinsky, MD[a], Michael V. Krasnokutsky, MD[a],
Michael Augustin, MD[b], Roland Bammer, PhD[a],*

- Degenerative disease and chronic instability
- Postoperative evaluation
- Trauma
- Infection and inflammation
- Ischemic/vascular injury
- Tumors

- Functional MR imaging in the spinal cord
- Nontraumatic vertebral body compression fractures
- High-field MR of the spine (3 T)
- Summary
- References

Over the past 20 years, imaging technology has revolutionized medical care, establishing radiologic evaluation as a vital part of patient management. General practitioners, and medical and surgical subspecialists, now rely heavily on imaging to establish and confirm diagnoses, and plan and monitor treatments. MR imaging is at the forefront of ever-changing and improving technology and has now become a practical and widely available tool for the diagnosis of a range of diseases. In the spine, MR imaging is the primary imaging modality for detecting disease because no other modality can provide the adequate contrast resolution necessary to differentiate the intraspinal soft tissue structures, and to reveal spinal cord or canal pathology. In addition, MR has proved to be the most sensitive tool for detecting infiltration of bone marrow [1]. Although the development of Multidetector CT (MDCT) has made major strides, affording rapid imaging and outstanding spatial resolution, its application to the spine has been limited thus far because of limited tissue contrast and artifacts from adjacent bones and surgical material.

Standard structural MR imaging sequences, including T1- and T2-weighted spin-echo (SE) and fast spin-echo (FSE), (spoiled) gradient-echo (GRE), and contrast-enhanced images, provide most of the information required for detecting and characterizing spinal pathology and achieving a differential diagnosis. Therefore, improvements to these basic sequences, generating greater tissue contrast, better spatial resolution, and decreased motion and susceptibility artifact, likely will provide the most significant gains in MR evaluation of spinal disease. As demonstrated in the brain, advanced techniques can provide additional information that increases the sensitivity and specificity of diagnosis, and more detailed physiologic or anatomic information that can help the referring clinician in guiding management. Diffusion-weighted (DW) imaging, diffusion tensor (DT) imaging and tractography, perfusion, MR spectroscopy, and functional MR imaging (fMR imaging) sequences are now often part of a routine workup in the brain for the assessment of strokes, tumors, and inflammatory lesions. Although equally promising for

[a] Stanford University, Department of Radiology, Lucas Center, PS08, 1201 Welch Road, Stanford, CA 94305-5488, USA
[b] Department of Radiology, Medical University of Graz, Auenbruggerplatz 9, 8036 Graz, Austria
* Corresponding author.
E-mail address: rbammer@stanford.edu (R. Bammer).

doi:10.1016/j.nic.2007.01.003
neuroimaging.theclinics.com

the diagnostic workup of spine patients, these techniques are seldom used in spine imaging because of the technical challenges that limit image quality, including the highly magnetically inhomogeneous material surrounding the spinal canal, the small size of the spinal structures, the relatively large craniocaudal extent of the spine, cerebrospinal fluid (CSF) and blood pulsation, respiration, swallowing, and bulk motion. In addition, a substantial amount of spine patients who would require radiologic workup have to be turned away or receive inadequate imaging results because of metal artifacts adjacent to the diagnostically relevant regions.

Advances in spinal imaging depend on improvements in both MR imaging hardware and software. In the last decade, spine MR imaging has benefited the most from the introduction of phased-array coil technology [2] and increased field strength, both of which increase the baseline signal-to-noise ratio (SNR) of a study, which is a major factor for successful spine studies that are notoriously SNR-deprived. With the recent advent of parallel imaging [3,4], multielement radio frequency (RF) coils have been improved and have enhanced the SNR of high-resolution MR imaging over a large cephalocaudal extent. With the availability of combined head and spine arrays, the entire spine can be imaged (either stepwise or by continuously moving the patient table) without repositioning the patient and changing the coil (Fig. 1). This advantage is of great relevance because often, the disease of a patient (eg, multiple sclerosis [MS] or neurofibromatosis) requires a total workup of the entire central nervous system and repositioning the patient is often tedious and associated with additional patient discomfort. In addition to the application of new contrast mechanisms and functional studies, structural imaging sequences have matured further, providing better SNR and spatial resolution within dramatically shortened imaging times. Similar to MDCT, there is a new trend toward volumetric acquisition of spine MR imaging data on the horizon, which will afford multiplanar or curved-planar reformations (Fig. 2).

Although "cutting-edge" technology often implies that the technology being developed is not available readily to every user or is still under investigation, most of the sequences discussed are, in fact, currently or soon to be available from most MR imaging vendors and could be implemented in typical radiology practices. The techniques discussed can be supported at a field strength of 1.5 T, but their usefulness at 3 T makes them more popular in clinical settings, so they could be incorporated into routine protocols. The authors describe these advanced sequences in the context of common clinical scenarios, and address how such

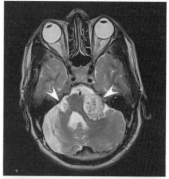

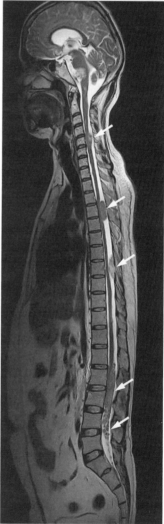

Fig. 1. Sagittal T2-weighted FSE of the entire spine and axial T2-weighted FSE through the skull base in a patient with neurofibromatosis type 2. Bilateral masses in cerebello-pontine angles (*arrowheads*) and throughout the spine (*arrows*) are clearly visible. New multicoil technology affords seamless imaging of the entire central nervous system without repositioning the patient. (*Courtesy of* G. Krueger, PhD, and C. Mohr, PhD, Erlangen, Germany.)

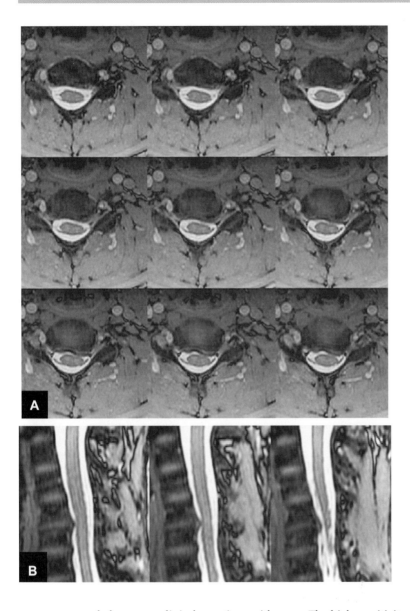

Fig. 2. Axial views from a modified 3-D balanced SSFP (COSMIC) scan of the cervical spine (*A*) and sagittal reformats (*B*). The interface between CSF and cord is well-identified, with superb visualization of nerve roots. Gray and white matter conspicuity is improved over T2-weighted FSE and GRE sequences.

sequences may help answer clinical questions with greater accuracy and precision.

Degenerative disease and chronic instability

One of the most common indications for spine imaging is the evaluation of back pain and radicular symptoms caused by degenerative disc disease and facet arthropathy [5]. The established role of MR imaging in this clinical setting is to identify the causes of the nerve root compression (including disc protrusions, osteophytes, and synovial cysts) and to assess the severity of spinal stenosis, and to exclude other conditions, such as infection and neoplasm, which may not be suspected clinically [6].

The high sensitivity of MR imaging studies is important because additional invasive testing, such as nerve root and facet blocks or discography, may be required in cases where standard MR imaging sequences fail to reveal a specific source of pain. Improved SNR with imaging at 3 T (Fig. 3), and decreased CSF pulsation artifact and improved spatial and contrast resolution using the new pulse sequences described below are likely to improve sensitivity for identifying subtle abnormalities. Such advances will provide the greatest advantage in the cervical spine, where small disc spaces and the relative paucity of epidural fat make delineation of disc protrusions more challenging than in the thoracic and lumbar spine.

In addition to identifying a possible source of back pain and radicular symptoms, referring

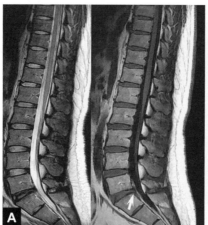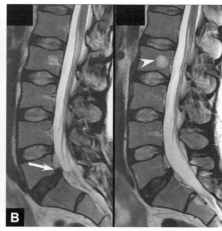

Fig. 3. 3 T Imaging. (*A*) Sagittal T2-weighted (*left*) and T1-weighted (*right*) images demonstrate relatively normal spine with mild degenerative changes of the L5-S1 disc (*arrow*). (*B*) Sagittal T2-weighted image of the lumbar spine demonstrates hemangioma at L2 (*arrowhead*) and a mildly protruded disc at L5-S1 (*arrow*) on T2-weighted scans. In both patients, the better resolution afforded by the higher SNR at 3 T allows for better delineation of the conus, anatomy of the vertebral bodies, and discs.

clinicians also look to MR imaging findings to guide surgical intervention. Detailed information regarding spinal canal stenosis, neural foraminal narrowing, and compression of nerve roots and the spinal cord can tip the balance in favor of surgical, rather than conservative, treatment. The identification of an extruded or sequestered disc fragment is vital information for the surgeon before intervention. MR imaging findings must be interpreted together with clinical information because symptomatic lesions cannot always be differentiated from asymptomatic lesions purely on the basis of imaging [7,8]. However, accurate delineation of the contents of the spinal canal and neural foramina may improve the diagnostic yield of MR imaging. Lesions that are associated with nerve root compression are more likely to be symptomatic, and therefore improved visualization of individual nerve roots and surrounding CSF, and more accurate assessment of the caliber of the spinal canal and neural foramina, are likely to improve the correlation of MR findings with treatment outcomes and help guide appropriate therapy [9].

For practical purposes, a short standard protocol, including sagittal T1- and T2-weighted sequences and axial GRE or T2, is desirable for screening the large number of patients referred for back pain. Improving the speed of these acquisitions with parallel imaging [3,4] is helpful not only to improve patient throughput but also to minimize discomfort for patients who suffer back pain and may have difficulty lying in a fixed position for long periods of time. In short, parallel imaging uses multiple small coils that are part of a phased-array coil, each of which has a different signal reception characteristic, to provide complementary image encoding through coil sensitivity, in addition to regular gradient encoding [10].

Axial GRE is used typically to assess degenerative disease in the cervical spine. Unlike with SE and FSE sequences (also known as turbo spin-echo), disc material (which is hyperintense on GRE) and osteophytes (which are hypointense) usually can be differentiated with GRE, regardless of flip angle [11]. In addition, the small size of the cervical disc spaces requires the use of contiguous slices, which is less feasible with FSE or SE. However, GRE often suffers from limited gray matter/white matter contrast and contrast to visualize nerve roots and foraminal stenoses better. Recently, a GRE method with multiple bipolar GRE formations has been introduced that combines the signal from the individual echoes. Here, early echoes provide increased SNR, and later echoes boost contrast (Fig. 4). This sequence type is known as Multiple Echo Recombined Gradient Echo (MERGE) or Multi Echo Data Image Combination (MEDIC) and can be performed as either a 2-D or a 3-D sequence. For the cervical spine, typical scan parameters are as follows: 650 ms/27 ms repetition time/echo time, 4 mm section thickness, 16 cm field of view, 512 matrix, 2 × parallel imaging acceleration. Three-dimensional imaging confers an extra advantage in the cervical spine, enabling sagittal oblique reformats to be generated that can demonstrate the obliquely oriented cervical neural foramina en face.

Balanced steady-state free precession (bSSFP) sequences also have an inherently high contrast between tissue and fluid. Moreover, compared with unbalanced steady-state free precession (SSFP)

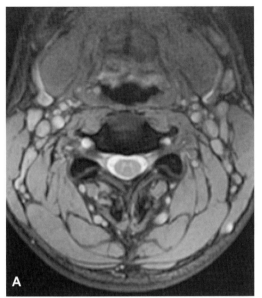

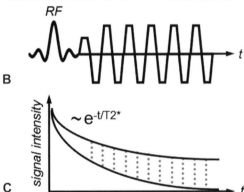

Fig. 4. Axial MERGE image of the cervical spine demonstrates excellent gray/white contrast in the spinal cord and good contrast between CSF and the cord (*A*). The good SNR and contrast helps demonstrate nerve roots extremely well. MERGE acquires multiple echoes during an oscillatory GRE readout (*B*), which become increasingly T2*-weighted (*C*). The echoes are combined in a way that the early echoes provide increased SNR, whereas the later improve contrast.

sequences (ie, the net gradient area within one repetition time (TR) is not zero), bSSFP provides high baseline SNR. Thus, it provides an efficient alternative sequence for better detection of herniations, sequestrations, or nerve root compression. Conversely, the gray matter/white matter contrast of conventional bSSFP is relatively poor. Modifications to the sequence, specifically ramping the flip angles up and down to increase contrast and SNR, have been suggested under the name Coherent Oscillatory State acquisition for the Manipulation of Image Contrast (COSMIC) (see Fig. 2).

SE and FSE sequences provide good anatomic detail in spine imaging and are favored for the evaluation of spinal canal diameter and for the detection of spinal cord abnormalities, with less susceptibility artifact from bone and improved contrast between gray and white matter structures within the cord, compared with GRE. Given the abundance of epidural fat within the lumbar spine, and the relatively large disc spaces, FSE sequences are favored over GRE in the lumbar spine to assess for focal disc protrusions and nerve root compression. However, the CSF adjacent to the cord, together with cord motion, often causes ghosting artifacts in conventional Cartesian imaging, and is particularly problematic in FSE T2-weighted images. Such artifacts create a substantial challenge for the radiologist in identifying small structures, such as nerve roots, within the CSF space. Radial sampling, in particular when combined with PROPELLER-type [12] acquisitions, is less sensitive to these types of distortions and improves the diagnostic quality of such sequences (Fig. 5). Recently, this method has been combined with fast-recovery (FR)-FSE sequences [13]. The benefit of FR-FSE over conventional FSE is the dramatically reduced TR, at similar, or even improved, T2 contrast between tissue and fluids [14]. With FR-FSE, assuming that the transverse signal of tissue (short T2) has decayed away at the end of the FSE train, a negative 90° (echo reset) pulse orients spins with long T2 (eg, fluid) from the transverse plane back along the longitudinal direction, leading to a much faster recovery of long T2 components to the equilibrium signal and thus, better contrast between long and short T2 species. FR-FSE has demonstrated great usefulness also for 3-D acquisitions because the TR, and thus the imaging time, can be reduced substantially [14].

Additional sequences may be helpful in the face of persistent unexplained symptoms, or for more complex or specific questions about anatomy or the influence of patient position on alignment and stenoses. Contrast-enhanced T1-weighted images with fat saturation can reveal facet joint pathology, spondylolysis, spinal degenerative/inflammatory changes, and changes within the paraspinal muscles, which are not always evident on conventional imaging [15]. Some studies also suggest that MR performed with axial load may add sensitivity and specificity to the evaluation of spinal stenosis and nerve root compression [16,17]. Similarly, dynamic imaging, with patients positioned to reproduce symptoms, may improve the ability to identify significant lesions. Often, abnormalities are apparent only during weight bearing in the upright position, or by flexion or extension of the spine. Although weight bearing can be studied in certain interventional magnets that have enough aperture to allow the patients to sit in an upright position, flexion and extension or lateral flexion

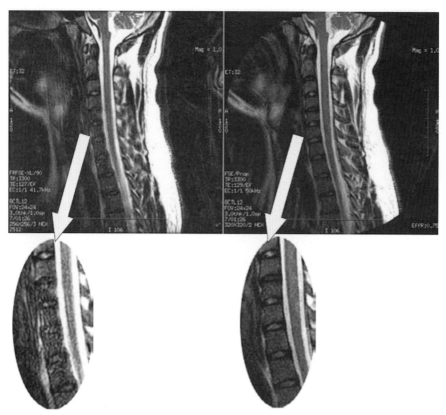

Fig. 5. Sagittal T2-weighted FSE with conventional Fourier encoding (*left*) and driven equilibrium T2-weighted fast-recovery FSE (FR-FSE) with PROPELLER readout (*right*). Conventional Fourier encoding is sensitive to pulsation and motion. Such artifacts demonstrate multiple ghosts along the phase encode direction (*left, see insert*). Because PROPELLER excessively oversamples the center of k-space with each PROPELLER blade, the pulsatile and motion distortions essentially are averaged out (*right, see insert*). (*Courtesy of* A. Gaddipati, PhD, Waukesha, WI.)

can be also accomplished in conventional magnets by using specific positional devices that allow different degrees of flexion/extension (Fig. 6). Certainly, great care has to be exercised when applying these maneuvers, and the selection of patients who might qualify for these kinds of tests should be made only with the referring orthopedic surgeon or neurologist.

MR imaging may provide important prognostic information regarding the potential for recovery following decompressive surgery in patients with long-standing myelopathic symptoms. High signal within the compressed cord on conventional T2-weighted sequences is nonspecific, representing a combination of myelopathic changes and surrounding edema. DW imaging may provide greater specificity than conventional sequences regarding which changes in the cord are irreversible. DW imaging is an MR technique that is sensitive to the random motion of water molecules in tissues over microscopic distances, and it can generate a map of the average apparent diffusion coefficient (ADC). Reduced ADC is seen in acute cerebral

stroke and aids early detection of infarcts, improving accuracy over conventional MR imaging. DW imaging also has become an invaluable technique for assessing other intracranial diseases, with applications in infection, tumors, and cysts. In one of the authors' studies [18], they found that spondylotic myelopathy presented with reduced ADC values, whereas the surrounding cord demonstrated elevated diffusivity. Presumably, the former is caused by either cord compression or vascular compromise, whereas the latter is caused by surrounding edema.

Postoperative evaluation

The challenge presented to radiologists by the postoperative spine is twofold:

1. Metallic surgical implants may produce artifacts that obscure anatomic detail.
2. Postsurgical reactive inflammatory changes can be difficult to distinguish from residual or recurrent disease or postsurgical complications such as abscess or seroma.

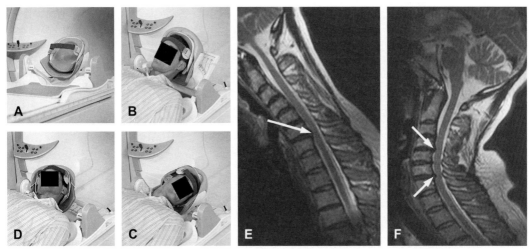

Fig. 6. Positional device (*A–D*) to anterior/posterior (*B*) or left/right (*C*) flex and rotate (*D*) a patient's head and keep it in the desired position for scanning. By performing scans in different head positions, such as anterior flexion (*E*) or posterior flexion (*F*), bulging discs (*arrows*) can be detected that may appear as normal in a neutral position of the neck. Such positional devices allow for an optimal assessment of spinal canal stenosis and neuroforaminal narrowing, improving correlation between imaging findings and clinical symptoms, because patients may experience pain only in certain positions. (*Courtesy of* G. Krueger, PhD, and C. Mohr, PhD, Erlangen, Germany.)

Metal in the area being imaged is problematic for both CT and MR. The concern for MR is the significant susceptibility distortions caused by the metal adjacent to the tissue. Although the metal itself cannot be imaged, these susceptibility changes in the proximity of the metal (eg, pedicle screws, metal fixation rods, metal cages, or endplates of artificial discs, and so forth) can lead to geometric distortions and signal loss or pile-up. Signal loss and geometric distortions can be reduced by smaller voxel sizes or thinner slices and excessive RF refocusing. Recently, new variants of 3-D FSE sequences (FSE-XETA, T2-SPACE, VISTA) have been introduced that differ from conventional FSE sequences by their excessively long FSE readout (Table 1). Here, a readout train comprises up to 200 echoes obtained at a minimum echo spacing, and allows image formation very rapidly, altogether diminishing artifacts (Fig. 7). A specific hallmark of these sequences is the flip angle modulation during the FSE readout. Here, the focus is to carry along magnetization as long as possible to avoid blurring and to provide optimal signal at the effective echo time (TE), ie, when the center k-space lines are acquired (Fig. 8). Using that regime, the specific absorption rate can also be diminished substantially. The volume acquisition follows a new trend that has been carried over from MDCT. By acquiring high-resolution 3-D volumes and subsequently generating multiplanar reformats or even curved-planar reformats, imaging could be made much more efficient. However, it remains to be shown whether these reformats are of sufficient quality and detail to replace additional, conventional cuts. By additional modification to the pulse sequence, different contrast and better gray/white differentiation can be achieved (Fig. 9).

Gadolinium-enhanced imaging is vital after surgery. Enhancement identifies areas of inflammatory postsurgical change, and recurrence of disease. Following diskectomy, recurrent disc protrusions are identified by their lack of contrast enhancement in comparison to uniformly enhancing scar tissue. After tumor resection, non-neoplastic enhancement can develop quickly because of postsurgical inflammation and neovascularity, and has been described even within the first 24 hours of brain surgery [19]. Early imaging following tumor resection maximizes the radiologist's ability to distinguish a residual enhancing tumor from postsurgical changes, and helps establish a postoperative baseline for the

Table 1: Acronyms of new pulse sequences

Pulse sequence	Vendor		
	GE	Philips	Siemens
Multiecho gradient echo acquisition	MERGE	—	MEDIC
Volumetric FSE	FSE-XETA	VISTA	SPACE

Other vendors might have similar sequences but these were not known to the authors at the time this article was written.

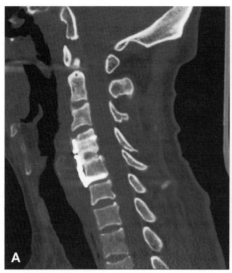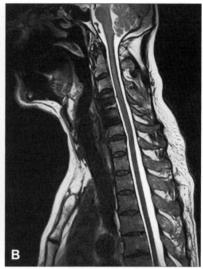

Fig. 7. (*A*) Sagittal CT reformation of the cervical spine in a patient with C4-5 anterior cervical disc fusion. (*B*) The new volumetric FSE sequences (FSE-XETA, VISTA, SPACE) afford much smaller voxel sizes and thus less intravoxel dephasing, improving MR imaging in the presence of metal, which typically is problematic because of the field perturbations created by the metal. That improvement, in combination with short echo spacing and excessive RF refocusing, dramatically reduces distortions in the spine, even in the presence of surgical hardware. (*Courtesy of* A. Ripart, PhD, Erlangen, Germany, and F. Ricolfi, MD, Dijon, France.)

patient. In on-going tumor surveillance, it is important to have high-quality, fat-saturated enhanced images to be able to identify areas of subtle new nodular enhancement representing tumor on the background of postsurgical scarring. Homogeneous fat saturation is critical when obtaining contrast-

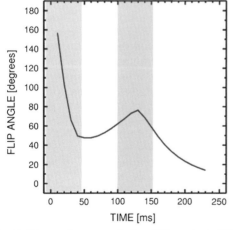

Fig. 8. Flip angle sweep during FSE readout. With high flip angles, the signal in FSE readouts is determined primarily by the primary echoes, whereas with lower flip angles, the signal becomes dominated increasingly by higher order echoes and stimulated echoes. To maximize signal for long echo train lengths, the flip angle of the refocusing pulses are ramped down continuously and raised slightly when the center of k-space is acquired to optimize contrast and SNR.

enhanced T1-weighted images, to avoid obscuring enhancement with signal from epidural fat and fatty vertebral body marrow.

Often, because of the harsh magnetic environment in and around the spine, or because of the presence of surgical material, frequency-selective, fat-suppression techniques or spectrally-selective excitation pulses are suboptimal (Fig. 10). Therefore, short-tau inversion recovery (STIR) techniques are used frequently, despite their obvious SNR penalty and the potential for altered contrast in the presence of contrast material. Recently, a variant of Dixon imaging has been introduced that has proved to be very robust (Fig. 11) and provides increased SNR [20] because of the combination of measurements. Especially for scans with number of excitations (NEX) greater than one, it appears to make sense to acquire data at slightly different echo times and to combine the data with the aforementioned iterative Dixon technique. One challenge for the Dixon method is too-rapid field fluctuations, causing the underlying phase maps needed for fat-water separations to fail.

DW imaging may be helpful in early postoperative follow-up as well. After surgery, patients may develop nonspecific fluid collections in the paraspinal soft tissues. Often, these represent seromas that will resolve gradually over time, with conservative management. Such benign collections do not demonstrate restricted diffusion, whereas frank pus within an abscess typically shows high signal on DW imaging, with reduced ADC [21]. DW imaging

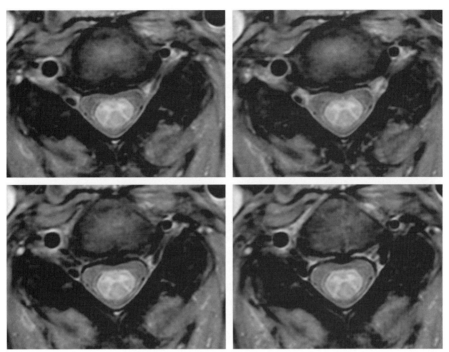

Fig. 9. Axial view of a volumetric proton-density–weighted FSE scan (VISTA) provides excellent gray/white matter contrast (*Courtesy of* F. Hoogenraad, PhD, Eindhoven, Netherlands.)

may be helpful also to distinguish ischemic injury to the paraspinal muscles from reactive enhancement caused by retraction during surgery [22].

Trauma

In the acute setting, CT is the primary imaging modality used to assess traumatic spine injury. CT of the entire spine with multiplanar reformats can be performed rapidly with high spatial resolution, and is much less sensitive than MR to patient motion. CT is more sensitive than MR imaging for the detection of cortical disruption caused by fractures, and can show subtle malalignment caused by subluxation of facets or vertebral bodies. MR imaging, however, can demonstrate ligamentous and cord injury, displaced disc fragments, and intraspinal hematomas not visible on CT, and not

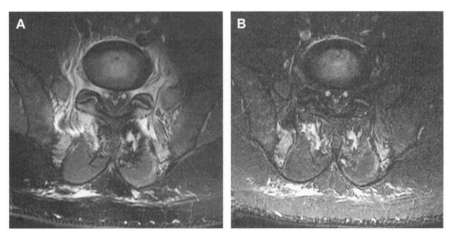

Fig. 10. Axial T2-weighted FSE images with spectral fat saturation (*A*) and short-tau inversion recovery (STIR) (*B*) in a patient with intrapedicular screws for posterior fusion (images below the screws). The geometric distortions from the titanium screws are apparent clearly on spectral fat saturation as increased signal in perivertebral soft tissues and in neural foramina. The field perturbations induced by the screws impair chemical fat saturation and lead to difficulties in separating fat from edema or fluid collections, which is significantly reduced on STIR.

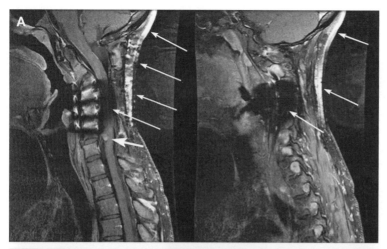

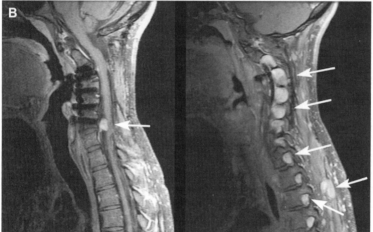

Fig. 11. Midline sagittal and parasagittal postcontrast T1-weighted fat-saturated SE images (*A*) and corresponding sagittal and parasagittal postcontrast T1-weighted IDEAL-FSE water images (*B*) in a patient with neurofibromatosis type 1 and spinal hardware. Numerous enhancing lesions are seen within the neural foramina (*large arrows*), abutting the spinal cord, and in the paraspinal soft tissues. The lesion adjacent to the spinal cord is visualized better in the IDEAL image (*B*), compared with the fat-saturated image (*A*), where failed fat saturation from severe B0 inhomogeneities from metallic hardware degrades signal in the spinal canal near this mass. Large areas of failed fat saturation (*small arrows*) show uniform suppression of fat in the IDEAL water images. (*Courtesy of* S. Reeder, MD, PhD, Madison, WI.)

infrequently is requested in a patient who has persistent neurologic deficit despite normal CT, or before treatment in a patient with abnormal CT findings.

A comprehensive MR imaging examination for spine trauma is demanding, requiring sequences that demonstrate anatomic detail to delineate ligamentous structures, disc spaces, and the spinal cord, and sequences that highlight edema indicating areas of acute injury. T2-weighted images with homogeneous fat saturation are key in imaging the trauma patient, because these demonstrate high signal extending through disc spaces and ligaments because of injury, and high signal from edema within vertebral bodies caused by microtrabecular fractures, without being obscured by high signal from fat. High-resolution T1- and T2-weighted images are critical in defining any focal disruption of the anterior and posterior longitudinal ligaments or the interspinal ligaments, and in identifying traumatic, sequestered disc fragments that may cause cord or nerve root compression, or

can become dislodged and cause neurologic injury if precautions are not taken during surgery. Focal areas of cord contusion and cord swelling are demonstrated best with axial T2-weighted images, but T2*GRE sequences are more sensitive to detecting hemorrhagic shear injury. Vascular injury may be suspected in some cases, and the addition of MR angiography and T1-weighted fat-saturated sequences may be needed to rule out arterial dissection.

Techniques that reduce scanning time and motion artifacts are critical to obtaining a complete and diagnostic MR examination. The authors described PROPELLER imaging with the FR-FSE sequence as a means of reducing image acquisition time and decreasing motion artifacts from CSF pulsation [13]. This method is also useful in decreasing artifacts from gross patient movement.

Accelerated data acquisition is a powerful method of decreasing study times and, consequently, reducing motion. Currently, parallel imaging offers at least a twofold to fourfold acceleration, relative to regular gradient encoding. Typically, the scan acceleration without significant residual reconstruction artifacts is limited by the number of coils, their arrangement, and their size, relative to the field of view. Here, parallel imaging capitalizes on the spatially inhomogeneous coil sensitivity profiles of individual coils that add additional image encoding to the regular gradient encoding. For 3-D sequences, acceleration applied to both phase encode directions (eg, reduction factor = 2 × 2) works better than if all acceleration is applied to a single direction (eg, reduction factor = 4). Parallel imaging methods, such as SENSE [3], GRAPPA [4] or any of its variants, can be applied to reduce scan time, to diminish blurring in FSE and echo-planar imaging (EPI) scans, and to reduce geometric distortions in EPI (eg, DW imaging) [10]. Parallel imaging has had a major role in the development and improvement of spine array coils, which afford imaging from the brain to the lumbar spine.

MR imaging can be challenging in trauma patients, not only because of poor patient cooperation and patient motion but also because of critical injuries requiring immobilization, the presence of fresh blood requiring universal precautions, and the necessity of monitoring equipment, which make repositioning extremely difficult. In trauma, more than in any other clinical application, it is therefore vital to be able to complete a comprehensive MR examination as quickly as possible without repositioning the patient.

Often, trauma patients have distracting orthopedic injuries or are unresponsive, and require imaging of the entire neural axis to rule out neurologic injury that is not apparent clinically. As mentioned earlier, the use of combined head and neck coils, in combination with moving table technology (including either stepwise or continuous table movement [23]), can facilitate imaging of the brain and spine without repositioning the patient or changing the coil, reducing the danger to the patient with multiple unstable injuries of being moved, and limiting the time the patient must be maintained in the poorly accessible environment of the magnet. The MR technologist is also protected from occupational injuries sustained while moving patients.

In addition to acute diagnosis, MR imaging is useful in the ongoing assessment and prognosis prediction of patients who have traumatic cord injury. Traumatic injury may result in cellular swelling and degeneration, the disruption of myelin membranes, or even more severe damage, causing functional deficits. Increased functional loss is also related to "secondary injury" [24], resulting in increased lesional size, swelling, and, ultimately, the additional degeneration of axonal fiber tracts. The exact stage of traumatic injury is often difficult to characterize by conventional MR imaging and it cannot detect possible therapeutic responses to neuroprotective drugs. Here, Wallerian degeneration above and below the site of injury is known to be indicative of axonal loss, but occurs only with advanced progression of tissue damage and is not differentiable from edema. It has been suggested that DW imaging might be able to define the type and extent of spinal cord injury better than conventional MR imaging, because different pathophysiologies may affect diffusion properties differently. In experimental animal models of spinal cord injury, a decrease of longitudinal ADC and an increase of transverse ADC were observed [25]. A spinal trauma can be complicated further if syringomyelia develops. In animal models, changes can be seen on ADC maps soon after 1 week, whereas conventional MR imaging is first positive only 4 weeks after the injury [26].

Infection and inflammation

A common role for urgent MR imaging of the spine is to rule out spinal infection, including epidural abscess and spondylitis/diskitis. Imaging of the entire spinal axis is recommended to assess for multiple sites of involvement [27], and the use of moving table technology is valuable in this setting. Contrast-enhanced T1-weighted images and T2-weighted STIR are helpful in identifying areas of active disease, but can be nonspecific. Enhancement with contrast material and T2-hyperintensity due to degenerative or inflammatory change may be mistaken for infection, leading to inappropriate treatment or the need for invasive procedures such as bone or soft tissue biopsy. As well, in the postsurgical patient, enhancement of scar tissue might be difficult to distinguish from enhancement due to infectious disease. High signal on DW imaging with reduced ADC has been demonstrated in spinal epidural abscesses and may be helpful to confirm the diagnosis of infection in the presence of an abscess [28]. Sequences such as 3-D COSMIC or MERGE may be helpful to assess involved structures because these provide superb intervertebral disc visualization. The presence of disc involvement may help to narrow a differential diagnosis of abnormalities further, and may favor infection over inflammatory or neoplastic causes in the correct clinical setting.

Inflammatory causes involve mostly the intramedullary space. Several inflammatory conditions affect the spine, with MS likely being the most common in adults. Although MS affects the brain in most cases, some patients present with only spinal lesions at the time of diagnosis. In these cases, imaging of the spine is particularly important if MS is suspected clinically.

For MS and for other inflammatory conditions, such as acute disseminated encephalomyelitis and nonspecific transverse myelitis, signal abnormalities visualized by conventional MR imaging are nonspecific and cannot be attributed to a particular cause. Therefore, the primary role of MR is to help detect a lesion, characterize its morphology, and determine its extent. Several studies have compared different pulse sequences and their ability to detect intramedullary lesions. Some studies conclude that fast STIR sequence is more sensitive than T2 FSE and magnetic transfer (MT) [29]; however, others find similar sensitivity between STIR and FSE [30]. The MT technique is used by some institutions because it may provide additional value in disorders affecting myelin integrity. MT imaging is based on the differences between "bound" water protons associated with macromolecules (proteins and cell membranes), and free, or "bulk," water protons and their respective pool exchange [31]. Either an off-resonant or on-resonant MT RF pulse can saturate the bound water protons, which, depending on the tissue's susceptibility to MT, leads to more or less signal reduction. Hence, the addition of an MT prepulse to a sequence (typically a T1-weighted sequence) can enhance the contrast between healthy and abnormal tissue. If the same sequence is repeated with, and without, MT pulses, the MT effect in tissue can be mapped as an MT ratio (MTR). The MTR has to be considered carefully because it can be confounded by various parameters, such as the type of MT pulse, continuous versus pulsed MT saturation, saturation efficacy, and so forth. Nevertheless, MTR can be seen as the logical next step toward a more quantitative MT imaging without taking the extra pain and going through true quantitative MT experiments [32].

Besides lesion detection, other morphologic parameters were shown to correlate with a patient's prognosis and disability, such as focal versus diffuse lesions (where diffuse abnormality correlated with a progressive, clinical course and greater disability [33]) and degree of spinal cord atrophy [34].

New advanced techniques described in this article may allow for better detection and characterization of signal abnormality within the cord by improving gray/white matter differentiation (VISTA and MERGE), reduction in CSF pulsation artifact (PROPELLER), and increased conspicuity between CSF and peripheral matter of the cord (FR-FSE). These techniques, combined with high-field MR imaging, provide for an excellent evaluation of inflammatory conditions. Essentially, the baseline SNR is doubled by 3 T MR; 3 T MR is especially important when imaging small structures such as the cord. Additionally, comprehensive imaging of the brain and total spine without repositioning shortens the examination time, and makes it more comfortable for patients who repeatedly undergo extensive MR imaging workups for evaluation of their disease.

Ischemic/vascular injury

Compared with ischemic events in the brain, ischemic cord injuries are relatively uncommon. Embolic or thrombotic events can be triggered by typical risk factors for stroke, and also by traumatic or interventional events, including spine surgery, vertebroplasty, or stenting. The most advanced technique in early diagnosis of ischemic tissues is DW imaging, which has been shown to be highly sensitive for the detection of hyperacute infarcts in the brain. Recently, similar findings were also reported for the spinal cord [25,26]. Although the number of subjects was very small in each of these studies, evidence is convincing that cord ischemia demonstrate a very similar characteristic on DW imaging as in the brain. The exact time course following the onset of cord ischemia, which should be considered when trying to determine the age of a lesion, is not yet known. Thus far, quantitative diffusion measurements in healthy volunteers confirm the assumption that diffusion coefficients in the spinal cord are comparable to those of the brain, and demonstrate diffusion anisotropy [35]. Despite the fact that DW imaging is well-established for imaging the brain, its use in the spine is limited, mostly because of the small size of the cord, CSF pulsation, and susceptibility artifacts induced by the magnetically inhomogeneous environment adjacent to the cord. Analogous to the brain, anisotropic diffusion is characterized most accurately by DT imaging [35], but DT imaging is challenged even more by the small cord size and motion.

To date, tissue-type plasminogen activator (tPA) treatment of cord ischemia is less common and, to the authors' knowledge, no study (except a case study [36]) currently exists that documents the efficacy or pharmacokinetics of intra-arterial or intravenous tPA for clot lysis in the spinal cord. An early diagnosis for early treatment initiation is therefore much less of an issue for spinal cord ischemia than for ischemia in the neurocranium. Rather, one is concerned here about ruling out other causes for stroke-like symptoms that would require alternative therapies, especially when conventional MR imaging is equivocal. Moreover, with conventional MR sequences, it may take days to observe intramedullary signal changes following spinal cord ischemia. Even then, it is often hard to discriminate such changes from those from other causes such as myelitis.

Aside from the lower incidence rates for cord ischemia, the small number of patients included in DW imaging studies of the cord also reflects the existing difficulties in applying DW imaging to the spinal cord in the routine clinical setting. The DW imaging technique most frequently available is DW single-shot EPI, which is notoriously difficult to apply to the spinal cord. Similar to conventional MR imaging, the small size of the spinal cord, the limited spatial resolution of EPI, and the adjacent CSF space sometimes make it difficult to quantify diffusion and to distinguish between gray and white matter. Improved imaging techniques, such as navigated interleaved EPI [37] or parallel imaging enhanced EPI [10], provide much better resolution and less artifacts than conventional EPI, and make the use of DW imaging in the spinal cord more relevant.

Most vascular anomalies of the spine are dural, arteriovenous fistulas, and arteriovenous malformations. Initial radiologic evaluation depends on the presenting symptoms, which are most commonly pain or neurologic deficit. Depending on the patient's demographics and the location of symptoms, cross-sectional imaging initially may be done to evaluate for degenerative changes such as disc disease and nerve root compression. Usually, MR imaging protocols for these purposes are done without the use of contrast and would not include MR angiography. In these cases, where no significant degenerative changes explain the patient's symptoms, a careful evaluation of spinal canal structures is appropriate for possible vascular anomaly. If no abnormality is seen in the intramedullary space and no obvious flow voids are present, careful attention should be paid to evaluating the extramedullary-intradural space for numerous tiny hypointensities that may represent flow voids in the presence of a dural AV fistula (Fig. 12), which are best appreciated on T2-weighted images. FSE T2-weighted sequences may have significant artifacts from CSF pulsation obscuring these flow voids; however, with the use of the PROPELLER FR-FSE [13] technique, the sensitivity of making this finding could be improved dramatically. Increased SNR on 3 T should be used to improve spatial resolution, which could help define the subarachnoid space further, in search of small flow voids.

Once the diagnosis of a vascular malformation is made or suspected on the basis of the initial study, further characterization should be made by angiography. Conventional angiogram is still performed at some point in the workup because it delineates vascular anatomy with the highest spatial resolution.

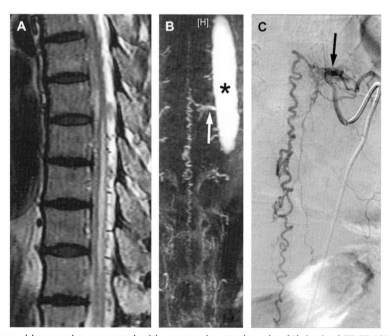

Fig. 12. A 70-year-old man who presented with progressive myelopathy. (*A*) Sagittal T2 FR-FSE images of the thoracic spine demonstrate edema within the thoracic cord. Multiple intradural serpiginous flow voids are seen, consistent with enlarged vascular channels. (*B*) Contrast-enhanced MR angiography with contrast bolus timed for maximal enhancement of the aortic arch was performed to evaluate for suspected dural AV fistula. maximum intensity projection reformats show the feeding artery arising from the left T8 intercostal artery (*arrow*) (Aorta is indicated by a star). (*C*) Digital subtraction spinal angiography confirmed the MR angiography findings (*arrow*) and embolization of the dural AV fistula was performed subsequently.

Additionally, it provides temporal resolution, making it possible to interrogate arterial supply, capillary phase and nidus, and venous drainage. However, it is an invasive procedure and requires the presence of interventional radiologists, nurses, technologists, and, sometimes, anesthesiologists.

MR angiography techniques have been improved dramatically to allow for better SNR, which allows the use of a larger matrix to improve the spatial resolution of small vessels within the spinal canal. Here, specific contrast-enhanced MR angiography (see Fig. 12) and 3 T might provide the conspicuity to characterize vascular malformations reliably. Specifically, 3 T offers increased baseline SNR and prolonged tissue T1 (relative to blood), which in turn boosts vascular contrast. Together with contrast agents with increased relaxivity and with better RF coils, this extra gain in contrast-to-noise might allow the appreciation of even very small vessels. Another noninvasive angiographic technique is CT angiography; however, it does not provide the distinction between arterial and venous structures that could be obtained from a time-resolved MR angiography, and is confounded in the spine by the presence of bone, which is not easy to eliminate during 3-D postprocessing of CT angiography images. Time-resolved MR angiography helps define the site of an arterio-venous fistula and resolve feeding arteries from dilated draining veins. The advantages of CT angiography, compared with conventional MR angiography, include increased spatial resolution and lack of artifacts that exist with an MR image, but cutting-edge MR angiography methods can compete easily with CT angiography, particularly when parallel imaging is added. The high baseline SNR of MR angiography is ideal for parallel imaging and enables one to speed up significantly the acquisition during the bolus passage, allowing better spatial resolution and arterio-venous separation. Here, the introduction of a recent contrast agent with shorter T1 relaxivity can provide even better vessel delineation for the same amount of contrast agent injected.

Tumors

MR imaging of spinal tumors is required not only for initial diagnosis but also for guiding therapy and monitoring the response to treatment. Classically, radiologists focus on localizing spinal lesions to extradural, extramedullary-intradural, and intramedullary compartments to generate an appropriate differential diagnosis, a surprisingly important step that highlights the importance of generating high quality T1- and T2-weighted images that are not degraded by patient motion or CSF pulsation and that have high spatial resolution. Extradural

neoplastic lesions are far more likely to be caused by secondary or metastatic disease, whereas primary lesions are more common than metastases in the intradural and intramedullary compartments. Primary lesions also differ between compartments, with lesions mainly arising from bone, muscle, fat, marrow, or notochord remnants occurring in the epidural compartment, and lesions arising from nerve roots, meninges, or neuronal or glial elements within the intradural and intramedullary spaces. Within their respective compartments, the exact location of lesions can be helpful as well. For example, identification of a lesion that surrounds or abuts a nerve root supports the diagnosis of a nerve sheath tumor. Diagnosis can be refined further if this lesion can be shown to envelop the adjacent nerve root, as occurs with neurofibromas but not schwannomas.

Sometimes, lesions transgress compartments, or the exact location of a lesion is difficult to resolve on MR images. In such cases, one relies on identifying some of the specific features that point to a specific location. Extradural lesions cause focal displacement of the thecal sac and its contents away from the mass. Extrinsic compression of the thecal sac occurs, and the CSF space between the lesion and the cord is decreased. Dura draped over the mass and an epidural fat-cap are helpful signs that one looks for on MR images to determine that a lesion is extradural. Intradural extramedullary lesions arise inside the dura, but outside the cord and cauda equina. These lesions tend to displace the spinal cord and enlarge the ipsilateral subarachnoid space with a sharp interface between the surface of the mass and the CSF space, creating a CSF-cap. Intramedullary lesions tend to expand the spinal cord, but may grow exophytically. Balanced SSFP sequences that have high contrast between tissue and fluid, including modifications to the sequence under the name COSMIC, the new volumetric FSE methods (FSE-XETA, SPACE, VISTA), or merely the better spatial resolution afforded by 3 T, as described previously, may be helpful particularly to characterize lesion location accurately in tricky cases.

Additional conventional imaging features may help favor one diagnosis over another, but rarely are definitive. For example, chordomas classically show bright signal on T2-weighted images with a low signal rim and septations, whereas lymphoma is characterized by relatively low T2 signal because of high cellularity [38,39]. However, such features are not definitive. Postgadolinium images improve the detection of intradural extramedullary disease and help characterize and delineate intramedullary lesions, distinguishing enhancing tumor from associated nonenhancing cysts and from the nonenhancing spinal cord [40,41]. In the postoperative setting, enhancement may be caused by either reactive changes, or residual or recurrent tumor. In tumors that involve the vertebrae or epidural space, effective uniform fat saturation is required because high signal from fat may otherwise obscure enhancing lesions.

Generally, the goals of new sequences in imaging spinal tumors are

1. To improve lesion detection and delineation
2. To differentiate different tumor histologies and grades
3. To separate residual/recurrent tumor from postsurgical and posttreatment changes with greater accuracy
4. To determine the proximity of lesions to key spinal cord tracts for surgical planning and prognostic information

Newer pulse sequences that have been investigated for use in spinal imaging have had mixed results. These include fluid-attenuation inversion recovery (FLAIR), T2w STIR, MR spectroscopy, DW imaging/DTI imaging, and fMR imaging. FLAIR is a heavily T2-weighted sequence that nulls signal from CSF and thus is expected to increase conspicuity of hyperintense lesions in close proximity to CSF. Despite its usefulness in brain imaging, FLAIR has been less successful in the spine, has been shown to be less sensitive than standard T2-weighted sequences in assessment of cord lesions [42–45], and is not recommended for tumor imaging. T2w STIR (a fat-suppressed T2-weighted sequence) is used commonly to assess for vertebral body involvement in the setting of trauma or infection caused by increased conspicuity of edema in the vertebral marrow, and may be helpful similarly in identifying vertebral body involvement with neoplastic disease, especially in poorly enhancing lesions. Despite several studies that have demonstrated increased sensitivity of STIR for cord disease in MS relative to other T2-weighted sequences [29,45], its application to intramedullary tumors may be limited by poor SNR and greater sensitivity to motion than standard T2-weighted sequences [43]. Fat demonstrates hyperintensity on FSE, which is caused by J-coupling. In certain cases, switching to true SE is a possible alternative.

Perhaps the greatest advantage of newer T2-weighted sequences in tumor imaging will be conferred by the reduced artifacts from patient motion and CSF pulsation, which will give a much more accurate visualization of lesions present within the cord and within the CSF space. This advantage can be critical when following patients for subtle changes in T2 signal that may indicate tumor recurrence, or when assessing intradural disease. In addition, as mentioned previously, SSFP sequences, including COSMIC, with high contrast between CSF and soft tissue, may provide a myelographic-type sequence that is effective for lesion localization and assessment of the intradural space.

In brain imaging, MR spectroscopy is used frequently to interrogate tumors. MR spectroscopy is a technique that can obtain biochemical information about tissues being studied by creating a spectrum of metabolites within a region of interest. Elevation of choline can be helpful in indicating increased cellular turnover and is therefore a marker of neoplastic disease rather than inflammatory disease, or posttreatment-related changes that can appear similar on T2-weighted sequences. As with all other methods, the small size and harsh magnetic environment of the spine pose a big challenge, but future advances may make this technique possible and useful in spinal cord imaging.

DW imaging, which can detect the altered cellular matrix of neoplastic tissues, may add to the staging of tumors and could help to differentiate different types of mass lesions. Promising results have been shown for the brain, where researchers reported DW imaging's ability to differentiate between cerebral tumor types; similar results might be anticipated for the spine. For example, in one patient suffering from an astrocytoma in the cervical cord, the authors found that the lesion had a significantly elevated ADC [18]. However, in high-grade, heterogeneous tumors, such as glioblastoma multiforme or high grade astrocytomas, ADC values can vary over a large range, and a general differentiation based on ADC can be difficult. Tumors with high cellularities, like lymphomas, usually demonstrate with massively decreased ADC. Also, abscesses and epidermoids present with hyperintensities on DW imagining because of restricted diffusion (Fig. 13), which ultimately makes the diagnosis.

Another approach is to use the orientation information obtained from DT imaging to perform fiber tracking, to determine whether a tumor invades or displaces fiber tracts. The displacement of fiber tracts might have consequences for the planning of surgical intervention and is currently the focus of several brain studies. Although fiber tracking is possible in the spine in the research setting, its accuracy has not been validated yet, and it is uncertain whether it will translate well to the clinical setting.

Functional MR imaging has been employed in brain tumor imaging to map out eloquent areas of the cortex to predict and minimize the morbidity of tumor resection by possibly limiting resection or altering the surgical approach. Such information is likely to be helpful in spine tumor imaging. However, at the current time, spinal fMR imaging still remains a research tool (see later discussion).

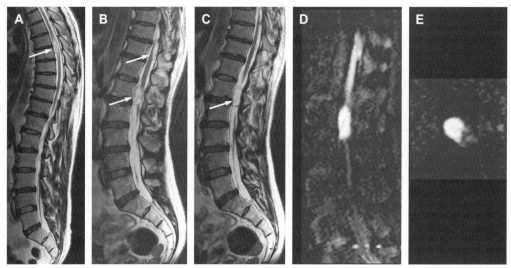

Fig. 13. Sagittal T2-weighted FSE images of the spine (*A–C*) demonstrate two nonspecific extramedullary-intradural masses requiring a differential diagnosis of several neoplastic causes. Sagittal and axial DW images (*D, E*) show these masses to have significantly reduced diffusion, thereby making a diagnosis of epidermoids. (*Courtesy of* M.M. Thurnher, MD, Vienna, Austria.)

Functional MR imaging in the spinal cord

The application of fMR imaging [46] to the spinal cord appears to be a logical extension to its cephalad cousin, but, in comparison, has received relatively little attention thus far. In addition to the usual challenges of obtaining high-quality fMR imaging data, the relatively low number of publications appears to be a consequence of the considerable challenge of acquiring MR images of the spinal cord. However, the urgent need for an fMR imaging method adapted for demonstrating function in the spinal cord arises from the fact that no other noninvasive, global method is available that can measure cord function. Because the cord is contained within the vertebral column, it is relatively inaccessible without opening the spinal canal and risking injury to the cord by inserting electrodes or needles and inflicting pain that could confound the study. The only means of assessing the function of the cord relies on the patient being able to feel a stimulus or having the proper reflexes. However, this method assumes that the sensory receptors, peripheral nerves, and relevant areas of the brain are all functioning normally. Even with normal function of these areas, very little information can be garnered about the cord's function distal to the location of an injury, and the relevant physical and physiologic information that may be needed for proper assessment of a patient's condition or the effectiveness of treatment is masked. Two possible options to improve diagnosis are fMR imaging and evoked potentials. With evoked potentials

(MEP, SEP, and so forth), one can allocate a lesion in the spinal cord and distinguish it from a peripheral lesion. However, it does not provide imaging information of activation in concert with structural imaging. Most challenges of spinal cord fMR imaging arise from differences in the magnetic environment among the bone, cartilage, and tissue [46]. The net effect is subtle magnetic field variations within these materials and field gradients at their boundaries, which can cause distortion and loss of signal. Respiration, cardiac, and CSF motion are other confounders that cause the field distortions to fluctuate rhythmically. After correcting for all these difficulties, Drs. Mackey and Glover at the authors' laboratory were able, for example, to demonstrate activation in the cervical/thoracic cord after presenting a nociceptive pain stimulus at the upper arm (Fig. 14).

Nontraumatic vertebral body compression fractures

Vertebral compression fractures in the absence of trauma are a common clinical problem in the elderly population. Although clinical history is helpful, up to one third of fractures in patients who have known primary malignancy are benign, and approximately one quarter of fractures in apparently osteopenic patients are caused by metastases [46]. Diagnosis of an underlying lesion is important because it influences clinical staging, treatment planning, and prognosis for the patient. In the chronic setting, the differentiation between pathologic

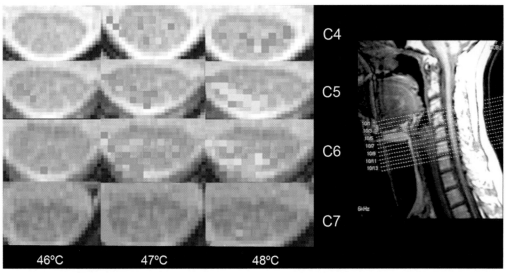

Fig. 14. Functional MR imaging in the cervical spinal cord during performance of nociceptive pain stimulation on the right upper extremity using a Peltier element to generate local heating. Clearly, activation increases with increased temperature of the Peltier element. To isolate the blood oxygen level dependent contrast effect, extra caution has to be exercised to minimize the influence from cord pulsation and respiratory artifacts. (*Courtesy of* S. Mackey, MD, PhD, and G.H. Glover, PhD, Stanford, CA.)

fracture due to underlying malignancy and benign osteoporotic fracture is fairly simple, and can be made with a high level of certainty [47,48]. Acute compression fractures, however, may share many of the imaging findings of metastatic lesions and differentiation is more challenging [49,50] Morphologic signs, such as complete replacement of vertebral marrow, involvement of the posterior elements, and epidural or paraspinal masses, can be used to improve the diagnostic accuracy in predicting metastatic disease, but may be equivocal. Results from recent studies have raised the hope that DW imaging might be able to differentiate benign from malignant acute vertebral fractures. It has been reasoned that proton diffusivity is elevated in osteoporotic fractures because of bone marrow edema. Conversely, metastatic lesions might change diffusivity only moderately, or even decrease it. It was postulated that a high cellularity of metastatic lesions, especially of actively growing tumors, would reduce proton diffusivity. Initial studies on DW imaging of the osseous spine to separate benign compression fractures from metastatic lesions were performed with a rather "exotic" DW SSFP sequence that is notoriously sensitive to confounders (eg, relaxation times, B1 field, and so forth) and that has an impressive discrimination capacity. However, subsequent studies using the more established Stejskal-Tanner–based approach reported less enthusiastic and more mixed results. To date, the diagnostic usefulness of DW imaging to differentiate acute compression fractures is still controversial. MR perfusion curves have received some interest, and a pattern of rapid wash-in and wash-out of contrast may be predictive of metastatic compression fractures rather than benign compression fracture [51]. In-phase and out-of-phase GRE imaging, which has been used for a long time to assess adrenal lesions in body imaging, is perhaps the most promising new technique suggested for the separation of metastatic spread from acute osteoporotic fractures. The use of in-phase and out-of-phase imaging to differentiate benign and malignant lesions is based on the assumption that malignant lesions completely replace vertebral body fat, whereas in benign lesions, fat is still present. Recently, Erly and colleagues [52] showed that a signal intensity ratio for in- and out-of-phase images of greater than 0.8 was able to predict metastatic disease, whereas a ratio of less than 0.8 could predict benign compression fractures.

High-field MR of the spine (3 T)

As mentioned previously, high-field imaging of the spine is appealing because 3 T MR imaging essentially doubles the baseline SNR, which can help when imaging small structures such as the cord, or using sequences that require rapid-acquisition, such as MR angiography. Issues that have to be addressed when migrating to high-field MR imaging are increased SAR and stronger sensitivity to susceptibility distortions. T2-weighted-FSE scanning currently achieves outstanding imaging quality;

however, there are still some unsolved issues with reduced T1 contrast at higher field and increased pulsation artifacts. Although the spectrum of T1 values widens with increased field strengths, many radiologist complain about the shallow T1 contrast at 3 T. A simple remedy is to change the flip angle from 90° to improve contrast, but by doing that, the SNR benefit is partially lost [53]. At higher field strength, the T1 relaxation times of semisolid tissue increases, thus requiring longer TRs to relax fully. CSF, on the other hand, does not change much, which has to be considered as well, especially when setting up FLAIR sequences.

Summary

The size and extent of the spinal cord pose a substantial challenge to the process of MR image formation in this area. Although similar contrast parameters as in the brain can be used for diagnostic workup, new sequences tailored to spine imaging provide better results than adapting conventional pulse sequences. In addition, more emphasis has to be placed on SNR and pulsation. During the last few years, major strides have been made in the development of new structural imaging sequences. The usefulness of more advanced methods, such as perfusion, diffusion, functional, and spectroscopic imaging, still needs to be shown. For many of these methods, further development in hardware and software is needed before such an assessment can be made, so that a method is not rejected prematurely.

References

[1] Ghanem N, Uhl M, Brink I, et al. Diagnostic value of MRI in comparison to scintigraphy, PET, MS-CT and PET/CT for the detection of metastases to bone. Eur J Radiol 2005;55:41–55.

[2] Roemer PB, Edelstein WA, Hayes CE, et al. The NMR phased array. Magn Reson Med 1990; 16(2):192–225.

[3] Pruessmann KP, Weiger M, Scheidegger MB, et al. SENSE: sensitivity encoding for fast MRI. Magn Reson Med 1999;42(5):952–62.

[4] Griswold MA, Jakob PM, Heidemann RM, et al. Generalized autocalibrating partially parallel acquisitions (GRAPPA). Magn Reson Med 2002; 47(6):1202–10.

[5] Hollingworth W, Todd CJ, Bell MI, et al. The diagnosis and therapeutic impact of MRI: an observational multi-centre study. Clin Radiol 2000;55: 825–31.

[6] Saal JS. General principles of diagnostic testing as related to painful lumbar spine disorders: a critical appraisal of current diagnostic techniques. Spine 2002;27:2538–45.

[7] Jensen MC, Brant-Zawadzki MN, OBuchowski N, et al. Magnetic resonance imaging of the lumbar spine in people without back pain. N Engl J Med 1994;331:69–73.

[8] Beattie PF, Meyers SP, Stratford P, et al. Association between patient report of symptoms and anatomic impairment visible on lumbar magnetic resonance imaging. Spine 2000;25: 819–28.

[9] Pfirrmann CW, Dora C, Schmid M, et al. MR image-based grading of lumbar nerve root compromise due to disk herniation: reliability study with surgical correlation. Radiology 2004;230: 583–8.

[10] Bammer R, Schoenberg SO. Current concepts and advances in clinical parallel magnetic resonance imaging. Top Magn Reson Imaging 2004; 15(3):129–58.

[11] Yousem D, Atlas SW, Goldberg HI, et al. Degenerative narrowing of the cervical spine neural foramina: evaluation with high resolution 3D FT, gradient-echo MR imaging. AJNR Am J Neuroradiol 1991;12:229–36.

[12] Forbes KP, Pipe JG, Bird CR, et al. PROPELLER MRI: clinical testing of a novel technique forquantification and compensation of head motion. J Magn Reson Imaging 2001;14(3): 215–22.

[13] Gaddipati A, Kumar A, Peters R, et al. Motion robust T2-weighted imaging of C-spine with PROPELLER with fast recovery modification. Proceedings of the Annual Meeting of the International Society for Magnetic Resonance in Medicine, Seattle, WA 2006;14:3140.

[14] Melhem ER, Itoh R, Folkers PJ. Cervical spine: three-dimensional fast spin-echo MR imaging— improved recovery of longitudinal magnetization with driven equilibrium pulse. Radiology 2001;218(1):283–8.

[15] D'Aprile P, Tarantino A, Jinkins JR, et al. The value of fat saturation sequences and contrast medium administration in MRI of degenerative disease of the posterior/perispinal elements of the lumbosacral spine. Eur Radiol 2007;17(2): 523–31 [Epub 2006 May 30].

[16] Willen J, Danielson B, Gaulitz A. Dynamic effects on the lumbar spinal canal: axially loaded CT myelography and MRI in patients with sciatica and/or neurogenic claudication. Spine 1997; 22:2968–76.

[17] Danielson B, Willen J. Axially loaded magnetic resonance image of the lumbar spine in asymptomatic individuals. Spine 2001;26: 2601–6.

[18] Bammer R, Fazekas F, Augustin M, et al. Diffusion-weighted MR imaging of the spinal cord. AJNR Am J Neuroradiol 2000;21(3): 587–91.

[19] Henegar MM, Moran CJ, Silbergeld DL. Early postoperative magnetic resonance imaging following nonneoplastic cortical resection. J Neurosurg 1996;84:174–9.

[20] Reeder SB, Yu H, Johnson JW, et al. T1- and T2-weighted fast spin-echo imaging of the brachial plexus and cervical spine with IDEAL water-fat separation. J Magn Reson Imaging 2006;24(4): 825–32.

[21] Guo AC, Provencale JM, Cruz LCH Jr, et al. Cerebral abscesses: investigation using apparent diffusion coefficient maps. Neuroradiology 2001; 43:370–4.

[22] Stevens KJ, Spenciner DB, Griffiths KL, et al. Comparison of minimally invasive and conventional open posterolateral lumbar fusion using magnetic resonance imaging and retraction pressure studies. J Spinal Disord Tech 2006;19(2):77–86.

[23] Kruger DG, Riederer SJ, Grimm RC, et al. Continuously moving table data acquisition method for long FOV contrast-enhanced MRA and whole-body MRI. Magn Reson Med 2002; 47(2):224–31.

[24] Liu XZ, Xu XM, Hu R, et al. Neuronal and glial apoptosis after traumatic spinal cord injury. J Neurosci 1997;17:5395–406.

[25] Ford JC, Hackney DB, Alsop DC, et al. MRI characterization of diffusion coefficients in a rat spinal cord injury model. Magn Reson Med 1994; 31:488–94.

[26] Schwartz ED, Yezierski RP, Pattany PM, et al. Diffusion-weighted MR imaging in a rat model of syringomyelia after excitotoxic spinal cord injury. AJNR Am J Neuroradiol 1999;20: 1422–8.

[27] Solomou E, Maragkos M, Kotsarini C, et al. Multiple spinal epidural abscesses extending to the whole spinal canal. Magn Reson Imaging 2004; 22:747–50.

[28] Eastwood JD, Vollmer RT, Provenzale JM. Diffusion-weighted imaging in a patient with vertebral and epidural abscesses. AJNR Am J Neuroradiol 2002;23:496–8.

[29] Rocca MA, Mastronardo G, Horsfield MA, et al. Comparison of three MR sequences for the detection of the cervical cord lesions in patients with multiple sclerosis. AJNR Am J Neuroradiol 1999;20:1710–6.

[30] Thorpe JW, Kidd D, Moseley IF, et al. Spinal MRI in patients with suspected multiple sclerosis and negative brain MRI. Brain 1996;119: 709–14.

[31] Balaban RS, Ceckler LS. Magnetization transfer contrast in magnetic resonance imaging. Magn Reson Q 1992;8:116–37.

[32] Ramani A, Dalton C, Miller DH, et al. Precise estimation of fundamental in-vivo MT parameters in human brain in clinically feasible times. Magn Reson Imaging 2002;20:721–31.

[33] Lycklama A, Nijehold GJ, Barkhof F, Scheltens P, et al. MR of the spinal cord in multiple sclerosis: relation to clinical subtype and disability. AJNR Am J Neuroradiol 1997;18:1041–8.

[34] Losseff NA, Webb SL, O'Riordan JI, et al. Spinal cord atrophy and disability in multiple sclerosis.

A new reproducible and sensitive MRI method with potential to monitor disease progression. Brain 1996;119:701–8.

[35] Ries M, Jones RA, Dousset V, et al. Diffusion tensor MRI of the spinal cord. Magn Reson Med 2000;44(6):884–92.

[36] Restrepo L, Guttin JF. Acute spinal cord ischemia during aortography treated with intravenous thrombolytic therapy. Tex Heart Inst J 2006; 33(1):74–7.

[37] Butts K, de Crespigny A, Pauly JM, et al. Diffusion-weighted interleaved echo-planar imaging with a pair of orthogonal navigator echoes. Magn Reson Med 1996;35(5):763–70.

[38] Wippold FJ, Koeller KK, Smirniotopoulos JG. Clinical and imaging features of the cervical chordoma. AJR Am J Roentgenol 1999;172: 1423–6.

[39] Mulligan ME, McRae GA, Murphey MD. Imaging features of primary lymphoma of bone. AJR AM J Roentgenol 1999;173:1691–7.

[40] Sze G. Gadolinium-DTPA in the evaluation of intradural extramedullary spinal disease. AJR Am J Roentgenol 1988;150:911–21.

[41] Sze G, Krol G, Zimmermen RD, et al. Intramedullary disease of the spine: diagnosis using gadolinium-DTPA-enhanced MR imaging. AJR Am J Roentgenol 1988;151:1193–204.

[42] Ross JS. Newer sequences for spinal MR imaging: smorgasbord or succotash of acronyms? AJNR Am J Neuroradiol 1999;20: 361–73.

[43] Lowe GM. Magnetic resonance imaging of intramedullary spinal cord tumors. J Neurooncol 2000;47:195–210.

[44] Keiper MD, Grossman RI, Brunson JC, et al. The low sensitivity of fluid-attenuation inversion-recovery MR in the detection of multiple sclerosis of the spinal cord. AJNR Am J Neuroradiol 1997;18:1035–9.

[45] Hitmair K, Mallek R, Prayer D, et al. Spinal cord lesions in patients with multiple sclerosis: comparison of pulse sequences. AJNR Am J Neuroradiol 1996;17:1555–65.

[46] Ross JS, Brant-Zawadski M, Moore KR, et al. Diagnostic imaging: spine. Salt Lake City (UT): Amirsys Inc; 2004.

[47] Baker LL, Goodman SB, Perkash I, et al. Benign versus pathologic compression fractures of vertebral bodies: assessment with conventional spin-echo, chemical-shift and STIR MR imaging. Radiology 1990;174:495–502.

[48] An HS, Andreshak TG, Nguyen C, et al. Can we distinguish between benign vs malignant compression fractures of the spine by magnetic resonance imaging? Spine 1995;20: 1776–82.

[49] Rupp RE, Ebraheim NA, Coombs RJ. Magnetic resonance imaging differentiation of compression spine fractures or vertebral lesions caused by osteoporosis or tumour. Spine 1995;23:2499–503 [discussion: 2504].

[50] Yuh WT, Zachar CK, Barloon TJ, et al. Vertebral compression fractures: distinction between benign and malignant causes with MR imaging. Radiology 1989;172:215–8.

[51] Chen WT, Shih TT, Chen RC, et al. Blood perfusion of vertebral lesions evaluated with gadolinium-enhanced dynamic MRI: in comparison with compression fracture and metastasis. J Magn Reson Imaging 2002;15:308–14.

[52] Erly WK, Oh ES, Outwater EK. The utility of in-phase/opposed-phase imaging in differentiating malignancy from acute benign compression fractures of the spine. AJNR Am J Neuroradiol 2006; 27:1183–8.

[53] Schmitz BL, Gron G, Brausewetter F, et al. Enhancing gray-to-white matter contrast in 3T T1 spin-echo brain scans by optimizing flip angle. AJNR Am J Neuroradiol 2005;26(8):2000–4.

NEUROIMAGING
CLINICS
OF NORTH AMERICA

Neuroimag Clin N Am 17 (2007) 137–147

Diffusion Tensor Magnetic Resonance Imaging and Fiber Tracking in Spinal Cord Lesions: Current and Future Indications

Denis Ducreux, MD, PhD[a,b,*], Pierre Fillard, PhD[c], David Facon, MD[a], Augustin Ozanne, MD[a], Jean-François Lepeintre, MD[d], Jerome Renoux, MD[a], Marc Tadié, MD[d], Pierre Lasjaunias, MD, PhD[a]

Magnetic resonance (MR) imaging plays a major role in the diagnosis and follow-up of spinal cord lesions. The main objectives of spinal cord imaging are to detect and characterize lesions, to assess the feasibility of surgical resection, and to diagnose recurrences and complications of therapy. Conventional MR imaging using T1- and T2-weighted sequences (in spin or gradient echo) lacks sensitivity in detecting and characterizing cord lesions, such as multiple sclerosis or acute spinal cord infarction. In addition, in patients who have cord tumors, conventional sequences may not be able to clearly identify the transition between the tumor and the surrounding edema. In the brain, diffusion-weighted (DW) imaging is an established and reliable method that helps to detect and characterize such lesions, and diffusion tensor (DT) imaging is becoming an important technique to identify white matter tracts and the effects of different lesions on them. DW imaging and DT imaging are usually performed using echo planar sequences, which are sensitive to noise, motion, and susceptibility artifacts. These two caveats make it difficult to detect and characterize spinal cord lesions, particularly with DW imaging. In addition, the resolution of most currently clinically used DW imaging

[a] Department of Neuroradiology, CHU de Bicêtre, Paris XI University, 78 rue du Général Leclerc, 94270 Le Kremlin-Bicêtre, France
[b] LIMEC, INSERM UMR 788, Le Kremlin Bicêtre, France
[c] Asclepios Research Project, 2004 route des Lucioles - BP 93, 06902 Sophia Antipolis, France
[d] Department of Neurosurgery, CHU de Bicêtre, Paris XI University, 78 rue du Général Leclerc, 94270 Le Kremlin-Bicêtre, France
* Corresponding author.
E-mail address: denis.ducreux@bct.ap-hop-paris.fr (D. Ducreux).

sequences is not optimal to image structures as small as the spinal cord and its internal features. Better characterization of white matter lesions (and therefore many cord lesions) may be achieved using DT imaging, an MR technique that evaluates the movement of extracellular water molecules within white matter fibers and enables the reconstruction of three-dimensional images of white matter tracts using specialized fiber tracking (FT) algorithms [1–5].

Recently, several investigators have assessed the feasibility of performing spinal cord DT imaging studies [5–10]. DT imaging sequences with computation of fractional anisotropy (FA) are more sensitive than spin echo T2-weighted images in detecting intrinsic abnormalities in acute or chronic spinal cord compression [5,11]. In lesions that produce involvement of white matter fibers, it has also been reported that DT imaging with FT may help to define abnormal areas that are undetected on routine T2-weighted imaging [5]. In our experience, FA and FT maps derived from DT imaging computations may help neurosurgeons to better delineate spinal cord tumors and may contribute important information before tumor resection.

In this article, we review the different methods available to obtain DT imaging and FT in the spinal cord and their clinical applications. We discuss novel and dedicated spine FT programs and speculate about the future of DT imaging and FT in spinal cord imaging.

Diffusion tensor imaging and fiber tracking methods

Image acquisition

DT imaging may be reliably performed on 1.5 T MR imaging systems with actively shielded magnetic field gradients, but strong gradients are needed (≥ 30 mT/m) for optimal imaging. To decrease magnetic susceptibility artifacts intrinsic to echo planar DT imaging sequences, parallel imaging with the shortest echo time is desirable. The spinal cord is a small organ with less extracellular water than the brain. Consequently, small b values are required to prevent signal attenuation on DW imaging. SENSE or GRAPPA echo planar imaging or multishot fast spin echo sequences obtained with a b value of approximately 500 s/mm^2 are most advantageous because they reduce magnetic susceptibility artifacts and result in shorter acquisition times [12]. Several DT imaging gradient directions are needed, and theoretically more directions result in a better signal-to-noise ratio and better diffusion ellipsoids. Investigators have tested 6, 12, 25, and 55 directions and have concluded that the best compromise between acquisition time and image quality is achieved with 25 directions (http://www.research.att.com/~njas/electrons/). Data are then converted to the sagittal plane (resulting a more complete visualization of the spinal cord than in the axial plane) using a simple matrix rotation. Sagittal DT imaging sequences are most sensitive to water diffusivity along the main spinal cord axis. To decrease cerebrospinal fluid partial flow motion, cardiac gating may be used, especially for thoracic cord imaging, but it is not mandatory if saturation pulses are placed in the region of the heart.

Based on these observations, we performed our studies using sagittal, single–shot, spin echo, echo-planar parallel GRAPPA DT imaging with an acceleration factor of 2 and 25 noncollinear gradient directions with two b values ($b = 0$ and 500 s/mm^2) (field of view: 180 × 180 mm; image matrix: 128 × 128; 12 slices with a thickness of 3 mm, nominal voxel size: 1.4 × 1.4 × 3 mm, and TR/TE = 4600/83 ms). Acquisition time is slightly over 3 minutes per study, during which time the patients are asked to hold still and to try to avoid swallowing.

Other acquisition schemes exist (field of view: 200 mm; axial 2 mm slice thickness, and b value ~ 800 s/mm^2), but to our knowledge they fail to generate adequate FT images needed to visualize the white matter tracts in the spinal cord (Metens and Balleriaud, personal communication, 2005).

Image analysis

Image analysis is performed on a voxel-by-voxel basis using our dedicated software (DPTools; http://www.fmritools.org). Before performing the tensor estimation, an unwarping algorithm is applied to the DT imaging dataset to correct for distortions related to eddy currents induced by the large diffusion sensitizing gradients. This algorithm relies on a three-parameter distortion model including scale, shear, and linear translation in the phase-encoding direction [13]. Optimal parameters are assessed independently for each slice relative to the corresponding T2-weighted image by maximization of an entropy-related similarity measure called "mutual information" [14]. This algorithm has proven to be fast and reliable and is used in many brain applications. We adapted it to the spinal cord to decrease the distortions induced by the echo planar sequence. DT imaging acquisitions can be further processed without distortion corrections, but FA and FT maps may show artifacts in the edges of the field of view. After distortion correction, the diffusion tensor and subsequently the Eigen system (with Eigen values $\lambda 1$, λ_2, λ_3) is calculated on a voxel-by-voxel basis as described in the literature [15]. Thus, the DT imaging tensor field (Fig. 1), the

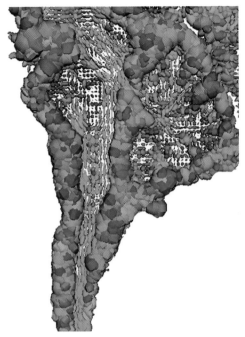

Fig. 1. Color-coded spinal cord DT imaging tensor fields using an ellipsoid scheme centered on the cranio-cervical area. Ellipsoids size and shape are related to the eigenvectors of the DT imaging acquisition. Large ellipsoids are seen in the CSF areas because its motion at a microscopical level is not clearly directional, resulting in a mixture of colors, shapes, and sizes. Conversely, the cord shows small longitudinal ellipsoids (mostly green and uniform in shape and size).

apparent diffusion coefficient (ADC) mean = $(\lambda_1 + \lambda_2 + \lambda_3)/3 = \lambda$, and the

$$FA = \sqrt{\frac{3}{2}} \cdot \frac{\sqrt{(\lambda_1 - \lambda)^2 + (\lambda_2 - \lambda)^2 + (\lambda_3 - \lambda)^2}}{\sqrt{\lambda_1^2 + \lambda_2^2 + \lambda_3^2}}$$

are calculated on the basis of formulas that incorporate the tensor elements to generate quantitative parametric ADC and FA maps. FA values of around 1 are nearly anisotropic, whereas FA values close to 0 are nearly isotropic.

Fiber tracking method

In addition to the two-dimensional parametric color maps (also called directionality maps) obtained using the previously mentioned method, three-dimensional white matter fiber tracts maps can be generated. These FT maps are based on similarities between neighboring voxels in the shape (quantitative diffusion anisotropy measures) and orientation (principal eigenvector map) of the diffusion ellipsoid (Fig. 1) [16–20]. Because factors

affecting the shape of the apparent diffusion tensor in the white matter include the density of fibers, the degree of myelination, the average diameter (beam) of the fibers, and the directional similarity of the fibers in a voxel, it is possible to access the fiber connectivity as previously reported [14,21–23]. The algorithm we recommend is based on extraction of the principal diffusion direction of the tensor field in the regions where the diffusivity is highly linear and a vector-based tracing scheme [24–27]. Other FT algorithms exist and are used in software packages provided by different manufactures or free of charge (dTV available at http://www.ut-radiology. umin.jp/people/masutani/, Brainvisa available at http://brainvisa.info, and DTI Studio available at: http://lbam.med.jhmi.edu/DTIuser/DTIuser.asp), but we believe that they fail to generate FT maps that are reliable for spinal cord anatomy. These algorithms are, however, appropriate for brain DT imaging studies. The algorithm we use was optimized to take into account the FA values in neighboring voxels in white matter tracts mostly oriented in the longitudinal plane (http://www-sop.inria.fr/epidaure/ personnel/Pierre.Fillard/). This occurs because water diffusion is greater in the "top to bottom axis when compared with that occurring in the transverse plane. The program estimates the tensor field of the DT imaging acquisition and then processes the entire study to find all detectable fibers. The user selects a region-of-interest that maps in three dimensions all fibers that pass through it. The process takes less than 30 seconds on a PC workstation.

Three-dimensional reconstructions of white matter tracts are color coded. Green denotes cranio-caudal fibers, blue denotes the left-to-right fibers, and red denotes the anterior-posterior fibers. FT reconstructions may falsely depict aberrant fibers that are due to susceptibility artifacts, especially in the edges of the field-of-view. These artifacts do not affect the intrinsic cord fibers and are easy to recognize.

Fractional anisotropy measurements

Spinal DT imaging can be used to generate three types of maps (similar to those used in brain DT imaging). In the directionality map, the fibers traveling in different directions (left to right, bottom to top, and anterior to posterior) are assigned different colors that permit their identification. These maps result in a two-dimensional display and contain important information regarding anatomy and anisotropy of white matter tracts. Unfortunately, their resolution is limited. Directionality and FT maps provide anatomic information but cannot provide objective values on FA. FA maps thus result in numeric information that may be useful in many disease processes. As with many other new techniques, we recommend that each center obtain a set of normal FA measurements that can be used for comparison in cases of lesions. Special attention should be paid to avoiding cerebrospinal fluid partial volume effects and magnetic susceptibility and motion artifacts in the selection of each region-of-interest (ROI). For example, we initially performed cord FA measurements in healthy volunteers at three different levels (cervical [C2–C5], high thoracic [T1–T6], and low thoracic [T7–T12]) using ROIs of 20 mm^2 (10 voxels), which included gray and white matter. FA values are nearly identical at the different spinal cord levels, implying that directionality of white matter fibers is remarkably uniform throughout the cord.

For spinal cord lesions, FA measurements should be performed at the site of abnormality using an ROI that is located completely within the lesion. To set the ROI, the b0 images are used because they permit clear visualization of the lesions. From them, these ROIs are copied to the FA maps to avoid partial volume effects and magnetic susceptibility and motion artifacts.

Clinical applications

Normal anatomy

FT of the spinal cord shows the main white matter tracts: posterior-lateral cortico-spinal, posterior lemniscal, and spinal-thalamic (Fig. 2). On the fiber tracking three-dimensional reconstructions, it is also possible to visualize the fibers of the nerve roots (Fig. 2).

Spinal cord tumors

DT imaging and FT may help to characterize some tumors and to delineate their margins [25]. FA values are similar for astrocytomas (0.48 ± 0.02), ependymomas (0.5 ± 0.04), and metastases (0.46 ± 0.04) but are different for hemangioblastomas (0.59). The lowest FA values are seen in metastases, and the highest are seen in hemangioblastomas. Because most tumors of the cord are gliomas, DT imaging may not play an important role in the histologic characterization of these tumors but may play a role in distinguishing hemangioblastomas from metastases (an observation that may be important in patients who have Von Hippel Lindau disease).

The margins of tumors as seen on DT imaging match those seen on T2-weighted sequences. Using FA maps, the surrounding edema may be separated from the tumor due to lower values in the former. FT may show fibers that are warped or frankly destroyed by tumor (Figs. 3 and 4). This may be important when assessing highly infiltrative tumors and delineating their margins before resection. In addition, tumors such as metastases and hemangioblastomas are localized and tend not to infiltrate the surrounding areas (Fig. 5). Rotation of the three-dimensional FT maps is needed in some patients to localize the tumors (Figs. 4 and 5).

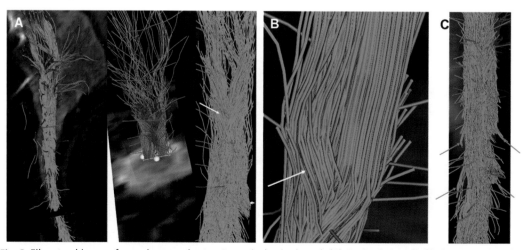

Fig. 2. Fiber tracking performed on a volunteer's cervical spinal cord. (*A*) Sagittal view (*left*) shows green color-coded posterior lemniscal tracts. A slightly oblique projection (*center*) shows the same tracts superimposed on an axial b = 0 image. Magnified view (*right*) shows the decussating fibers (*arrow*) of these tracts. (*B*) Magnified view shows decussation of the spino-thalamic tracts (*arrow*). (*C*) Frontal view of the cervical spine shows fibers in nerve roots (*arrows*).

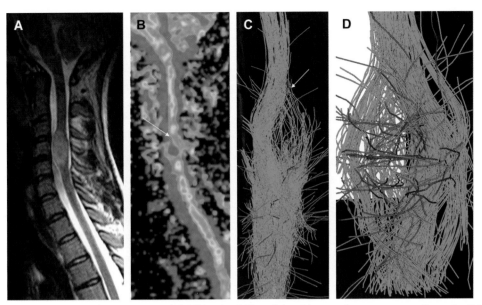

Fig. 3. Cervical spinal cord astrocytoma. (*A*) Midsagittal T2-weighted image shows an expansile and mildly hyperintense tumor at the C2–C4 levels. (*B*) Directionality sagittal map shows loss of anisotropy in the mass (*blue color, arrow*) that is focal and compatible with diagnosis of WHO grade II astrocytoma. Anisotropy is immediately reestablished along tumor margins due to the lack of edema. (*C*) FT map shows splaying of fibers by a tumor normalized at the tumor margin (*arrow*). (*D*) Magnified FT map shows fiber splaying by a tumor. Most fibers are intact due to the nondestructive nature of tumor.

Spinal cord compression

Conventional T2-weighted images may underestimate the effects of compressive lesions on the spinal cord, particularly when no hyperintense signal accompanies cord compression in the hyperacute period (which is the critical time to treat these lesions). DT imaging can detect abnormal areas within a normal-appearing spinal cord on

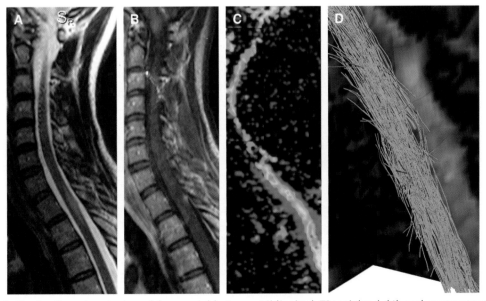

Fig. 4. Cervico-thoracic spinal cord hemangioblastoma. Midsagittal T2-weighted (*A*) and postcontrast T1-weighted images (*B*) show focal enhancing lesion on the posterior aspect of the cord at the T1 level with surrounding edema. (*C*) Directionality map shows focal loss of anisotropy (*blue color*) in this noninvasive tumor. Anisotropy recovers immediately outside of the tumor margins. (*D*) Oblique FT map shows the focal "hole" where the tumor is located. Note splaying of fibers but no significant thinning or invasion.

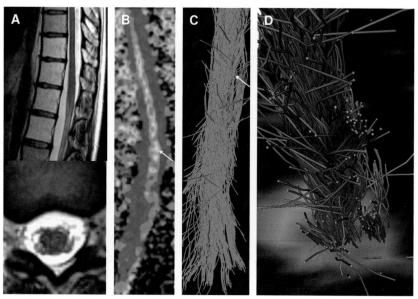

Fig. 5. Breast metastasis to the conus medullaris. (*A*) Midsagittal (*upper*) and axial (*lower*) T2-weighted image shows no significant abnormality. (*B*) Corresponding directionality map shows localized loss of anisotropy in this tumor. Metastases are well marginated tumors that generally do not invade the surrounding tissues. (*C*) Frontal FT map fails to show the lesion as a small "hole" (*arrow*) amid fibers. Note the nerve roots of the cauda equina inferiorly. (*D*) Oblique FT map shows to a better extent the focal hole corresponding to the site of the tumor in the inferior and left lateral aspect of the cord. Neighboring fibers are preserved. This case illustrates the significant sensitivity of DT imaging to localized lesions even when T2-weighted images are normal.

T2-weighted imaging. FA has a better sensitivity (73%) and specificity (100%) in the detection of acute spinal cord abnormalities compared with conventional T2-weighted imaging [5]. FA measurements versus the time of injury may also help to predict the patients' outcome (good outcome for FA values >0.6 and worse outcome for FA values <0.6 in the acute period) (Fig. 6). FT identifies the sites of compression and aids by depicting mass effect and discontinuity of white matter fibers, which also have a prognostic implication because patients who have the latter generally show little or no improvement (Fig. 7).

Myelitis

DT imaging is more sensitive than regular T2-weighted imaging in detecting spinal cord inflammatory lesions. FA maps and FT performed on patients who have suspected myelitis show lesions that are not seen on conventional T2 imaging. In one series, patients who had idiopathic myelitis had one (100%) or multiple (80%) areas of

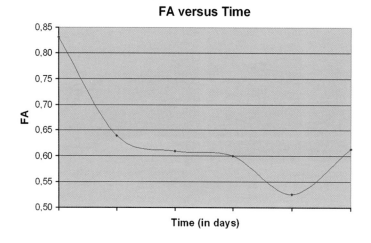

FA versus Time

Fig. 6. Time-course curve from Day 1 to Day 30 of the averaged FA estimated from sites of spinal cord compression. FA values decrease from Day 1 through Day 21 and then slightly increase. This phenomenon is related to extracellular water diffusivity. There is restricted diffusivity in the acute stage and increased diffusivity in the chronic stage. Preservation of diffusivity in the acute stage may imply a better prognosis.

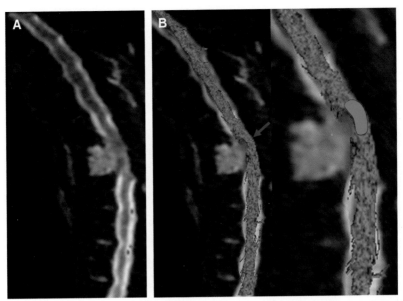

Fig. 7. Spinal cord compression due to vertebral and epidural metastasis of a breast cancer. (*A*) Midsagittal *b* = 0 image is shown on the left. (*B*) Color-coded FA map (red) shows a mass-effect on fiber tracts (*arrow*) but preserved anisotropy in this patient, who had pain but no neurologic symptoms.

decreased FA regardless of the appearance of the cord at those levels on T2-weighted imaging [12]. Increased FA may be seen in the periphery of the zone of myelitis and in normal-appearing T2-weighted areas. The latter zones tend to be asymptomatic; the significance of this finding is uncertain. Thus, an inflammatory myelitis is characterized by decreased FA values in the region of the T2-weighted lesion and increased FA values in the lesion's boundaries (Fig. 8). This pattern is different from that seen in invasive tumors, in which FA is low in peripheral regions of edema. Additionally, FT shows that inflammatory lesions spread the fibers of the spinal cord in areas that have an abnormal T2 signal; this pattern may be related to a decrease in extracellular water due to cytotoxic edema, axonal cluster regeneration, or cellular infiltration by inflammatory cells [28,29]. This pattern is not seen in invasive tumors and may be an important marker of inflammatory lesions. Occasionally, fiber thinning is seen in inflammatory lesions and may be due to early axonal involvement (Fig. 9).

Arteriovenous malformations

In spinal cord arteriovenous malformations, DT imaging with FA measurements may help to better understand their pathophysiology [30,31]. Additionally, FA values may improve after embolization and correlate with a better patient outcome. FT shows that at the level of the arteriovenous malformation nidus, the tracts are spread, shifted without spreading, interrupted, or normal. FT shows no

fibers running through the nidus, an observation that may become important if surgical resection is contemplated. Distant to the nidus, congestive edema or a "cavitation" pattern may be found. In congestive edema, FT shows spreading of fascicles with global enlargement of the beam of tracts.

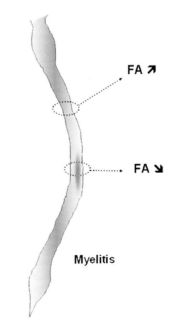

Fig. 8. Diagram illustrating FA variations seen in inflammatory myelitis. The centers of these lesions show decreased FA values, and their boundaries show increased FA. This pattern may be specific to myelitis.

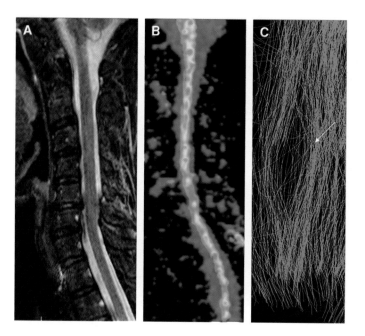

Fig. 9. Idiopathic inflammatory cervical myelopathy (presumed diagnosis). (*A*) Midsagittal T2-weighted image shows faint hyperintensity and expansion of the cord at the C5–C6 levels. (*B*) Corresponding directionality map shows loss of anisotropy greater than the size of the lesion seen on the T2 image. (*C*) FT map shows splaying and loss of fibers greater than that seen in localized tumors and due to the ill-defined nature of this inflammatory process, which resolves with antiinflammatory drugs.

There can also be a slight rarefaction of tracts, with decreased FA but normal ADC values. In cavitation, FT shows a loss of tracts with global thinning of their beam. Damage due to cavitation may be irreversible. In segments of the cord distant to the nidus without T2-weighted hyperintensity but where draining veins are present, FA values are slightly decreased when compared with segments where no draining veins are present, implying abnormal congestion at a microscopic level and perhaps

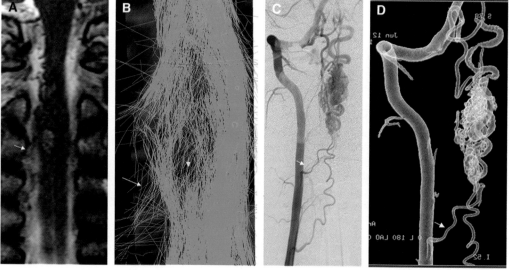

Fig. 10. Cervical spinal cord arteriovenous malformations in a 23-year-old man who had sensory symptoms in the right arm of 4 years duration. (*A*) Coronal T2-weighted image shows an intramedullary lesion at C3–C4 with an associated enlarged blood vessel laterally (*arrow*). (*B*) FT map shows segmental interruption of the right posterior fascicle (*arrowhead*) at the level of the inferior part of the arteriovenous malformation nidus, which also splays the fibers. Lateral fibers are interrupted, and nerve root fibers are thin (*arrow*). Frontal views of catheter angiogram (*C*) and three-dimensional reformation (*D*) from the catheter angiogram show the malformation. The arrow points to an inferior feeding artery that presumably resulted in alteration of nerve root fibers shown on the FT map. DT imaging findings suggest that the symptoms are associated with tract damage and that recovery of neurologic function may not occur after treatment. The zone of fiber disruption may be used for surgical approach to avoid further damage of intact fibers elsewhere.

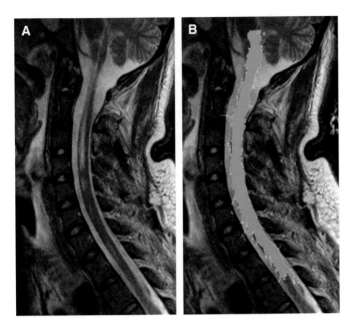

Fig. 11. A patient who has MELAS and spinal cord involvement. (*A*) Midsagittal T2-weighted image shows the central area of high signal in the cord from C2–C4. (*B*) FT map coregistered and projected on T2-weighted image shows an unaltered shape of the white matter tracts. In this disease, accumulation of extracellular water does not warp the fiber. In this map, the reconstructed fibers were subjectively assigned a red color.

explaining patients' symptoms when the level of edema seen on T2-weighted images does not match clinical deficits (Fig. 10).

Metabolic disorders

MELAS (mitochondrial encephalopathy, lactic acidosis, and stroke-like events) is a disorder that affects the brain and spinal cord. Patients who have spinal cord involvement have a worse prognosis. On the T2-weighted and FLAIR images, multiple, abnormal, high-intensity signal lesions may be seen in the mesencephalon, medulla oblongata, cerebellum, and cervical spinal cord. FA values are decreased within the spinal cord of these patients even when T2 abnormalities are not obvious [32].

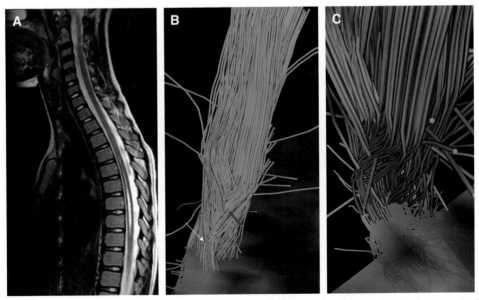

Fig. 12. Fluid-filled cavity in the thoracic spinal cord. (*A*) Midsagittal T2-weighted image shows syrinx in the lower thoracic cord. (*B*) FT map shows that the syrinx alters the shape of white matter fibers especially the spinothalamic tracts (*arrow*), which may explain symptoms in some patients. (*C*) Magnified FT map demonstrates the decussating tracts that are warped by the cavitation (*arrow*). Objective warping or tracts may lead to decompression even in patients who have small syrinxes.

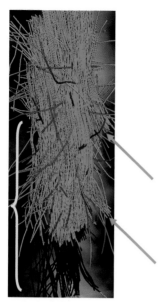

Fig. 13. A patient who has paraplegia after a spinal cord injury. Frontal view of the FT map shows a relative absence of right sided-fibers (*yellow bracket*) when compared with the opposite side due to Wallerian degeneration. Note the normal nerve roots (*arrows*), which are not identified in the area of Wallerian degeneration. The nerve roots on the opposite side could be used for a nerve bypass to the remaining functional spinal cord. The oblique FT map shows to a better advantage the scarce fibers (*yellow bracket*) due to Wallerian degeneration when compared with the normal side (*arrow*).

FT in the cervical spinal cord is not sensitive enough to detect abnormalities in MELAS patients. In MELAS, the extracellular water may not alter the shape of the tracts because the edema is not severe enough to warp them (Fig. 11) [32].

Syringomyelia

DT imaging may be useful to investigate syringomyelia. A syrinx may involve the spinothalamic tracts and result in temperature and sensory deficits and pain not directly related to the site and size of the lesion. Preliminary work in our laboratory seems to indicate that detailed anatomic evaluations in these patients are possible using FT. FT is useful in identifying the spinothalamic tracts in patients who have syrinx. We hypothesize that if the tracts are present but displaced by the lesion, the patients will have a better prognosis than when FT shows thinning or destruction of these tracts (Fig. 11). Identification of these tracts may be useful to the surgeon before placement of electrodes to control pain (Fig. 12).

Spinal cord injuries

Patients who have had prior spinal cord injuries may benefit from DT imaging and FT. Preliminary results after peripheral nerve grafting seem promising (Tadie, personal communication, 2002, [18]). Patients treated this way experienced a 40% motor recovery. Our early experience shows that FT may be used to assure the anatomic presence of intact fibers, a factor needed for successful grafting (Fig. 13). Fibers destroyed by the initial injury or secondarily to Wallerian degeneration do not respond to grafting.

Summary

DT imaging and FA may be more sensitive than other conventional MR imaging techniques to detect, characterize, and map the extent of spinal cord lesions. FT offers the possibility of visualizing the integrity of white matter tracts surrounding some lesions, and this indirect information may help in formulating a differential diagnosis and in planning biopsies or resection. FA measurements may also play a role in predicting the outcome of patients who have spinal cord lesions.

References

[1] LeBihan D. Molecular diffusion nuclear magnetic resonance imaging. Magn Reson Q 1991; 7:1–30.

[2] Basser P, Mattiello J, LeBihan D. MR diffusion tensor spectroscopy and imaging. Biophys J 1994; 66:259–67.

[3] Basser P, Pierpaoli C. Microstructural and physiological features of tissues elucidated by quantitative-diffusion-tensor. MRI. J Magn Reson 1996; 111:209–19.

[4] Wheeler-Kingshott C, Hickman S, Parker G, et al. Investigating cervical spinal cord structure using axial diffusion tensor imaging. Neuroimage 2002; 16:93–102.

[5] Facon D, Ozanne A, Fillard P, et al. MR diffusion tensor imaging and fiber tracking in spinal cord compression. AJNR Am J Neuroradiol 2005;26: 1587–94.

[6] Holder C, Muthupillai R, Mukundan S, et al. Diffusion-weighted MR imaging of the normal human spinal cord in vivo. AJNR Am J Neuroradiol 2000;21:1799–806.

[7] Ries M, Jones R, Dousset V, et al. Diffusion tensor MRI of the spinal cord. Magn Reson Med 2000; 44:884–92.

[8] Clark C, Werring D, Miller D. Diffusion imaging of the spinal cord in vivo: estimation of the principal diffusivities and application to multiple sclerosis. Magn Reson Med 2000;43:133–8.

[9] Bammer R, Fazekas F, Augustin M, et al. Diffusion-weighted MR imaging of the spinal cord. AJNR Am J Neuroradiol 2000;21:587–91.

[10] Cercignani M, Horsfield M, Agosta F, et al. Sensitivity-encoded diffusion tensor MR imaging of the cervical cord. AJNR Am J Neuroradiol 2003; 24:1254–6.

[11] Demir A, Ries M, Moonen C, et al. Diffusion-weighted MR imaging with apparent diffusion coefficient and apparent diffusion tensor maps in cervical spondylotic myelopathy. Radiology 2003;229:37–43.

[12] Renoux J, Facon D, Fillard P, et al. MR diffusion tensor imaging and fiber tracking in inflammatory diseases of the spinal cord. AJNR Am J Neuroradiol 2006;27(9):1947–51.

[13] Haselgrove JC, Moore JR. Correction of distortion of echo-planar images used to calculate the apparent diffusion coefficient. Magnetic Resonance in Medicine 1996;36:960–4.

[14] Poupon C, Clarck CA, Frouin V, et al. Regularization of diffusion-based direction maps for the tracking of brain white matter fascicles. Neuroimage 2000;12(2):184–95.

[15] Basser P, Mattiello J, LeBihan D. Estimation of the effective self-diffusion tensor from the NMR spin echo. J Magn Reson 1994;103:247–54.

[16] Ulug AM, Van Zijl PCM. Orientation-independent diffusion imaging without tensor diagonalization: anisotropy definition based on physical attributes of the diffusion ellipsoid. J Magn Reson Imaging 1999;9:804–13.

[17] Alexander AL, Hasan K, Kindlmann G, et al. A geometric analysis of diffusion tensor measurements of the human brain. Magn Reson Med 2000;44:283–91.

[18] Woods RP, Cherry SR, Mazziotta JC. Rapid automated algorithm for aligning and reslicing PET images. Journal of Computer Assisted Tomography 1992;16:620–33.

[19] Woods RP, Grafton ST, Holmes CJ, et al. Automated image registration: I. General methods and intrasubject, intramodality validation. Journal of Computer Assisted Tomography 1998; 22:141–54.

[20] Woods RP, Grafton ST, Watson JDG, et al. Automated image registration: II. Intersubject validation of linear and nonlinear models. Journal of Computer Assisted Tomography 1998;22: 155–65.

[21] Basser PJ. Fiber-tractography via diffusion tensor MRI (DTMRI). Proceedings for the VIth ISMRM Meeting. Sydney (Australia); 1998. p. 1226.

[22] Basser P, Pierpaoli C. A simplified method to measure the diffusion tensor from seven MR images. Magnetic Resonance in Medicine 1998;39: 928–34.

[23] Pierpaoli C, Basser PJ. Towards a quantitative assessment of diffusion anisotropy. Magn Reson Med 1996;36:893–906.

[24] Westin CF, Maier SE, Mamata H, et al. Processing and visualization for diffusion tensor MRI. Med Image Anal 2002;6:93–108.

[25] Xu D, Mori S, Solaiyappan M, et al. A framework for callosal fiber distribution analysis. Neuroimage 2002;17:1131–43.

[26] Elshafiey I, Bilgen M, He R, et al. In vivo diffusion tensor imaging of rat spinal cord at 7 T. Magn Reson Imaging 2002;20:243–7.

[27] Ducreux D, Lepeintre JF, Fillard P, et al. MR diffusion tensor imaging and fiber tracking in 5 spinal cord astrocytomas. AJNR Am J Neuroradiol 2006;27:214–6.

[28] Cassol E, Ranjeva JP, Berry I. Diffusion tensor imaging in multiple sclerosis: a tool for monitoring changes in normal-appearing white matter. Mult Scler 2004;10:188–96.

[29] Ciccarelli O, Werring DJ, Thompson AJ. A study of the mechanisms of normal-appearing white matter damage in multiple sclerosis using diffusion tensor imaging: evidence of Wallerian degeneration. J Neurol 2003;250:287–92.

[30] Ozanne A, Ducreux D, Facon D, et al. MR diffusion tensor imaging and fiber tracking in spinal cord arteriovenous malformations. AJNR Am J Neuroradiol, in press.

[31] Stein BM, McCormick PC. Intramedullary neoplasms and vascular malformations. Clin Neurosurg 1992;39:361–87.

[32] Ducreux D, Nasser G, Lacroix C, et al. MR diffusion tensor imaging, fiber tracking and single-voxel spectroscopy findings in an unusual MELAS case. AJNR Am J Neuroradiol 2005;26:1840–4.

NEUROIMAGING
CLINICS
OF NORTH AMERICA

Neuroimag Clin N Am 17 (2007) 149–152

Index

Note: Page numbers of article titles are in **boldface** type.

Moving?

Make sure your subscription moves with you!

To notify us of your new address, find your **Clinics Account Number** (located on your mailing label above your name), and contact customer service at:

E-mail: elspcs@elsevier.com

800-654-2452 (subscribers in the U.S. & Canada)
407-345-4000 (subscribers outside of the U.S. & Canada)

Fax number: 407-363-9661

Elsevier Periodicals Customer Service
6277 Sea Harbor Drive
Orlando, FL 32887-4800

*To ensure uninterrupted delivery of your subscription, please notify us at least 4 weeks in advance of move.